"With Solomon-like wisdom, Frances justly doles out blame and offers reasonable remedies. His decree: don't medicalize human difference; celebrate it."   —*Booklist* (starred review)

"Persuasive. . . . Authoritative."   —*American Scholar*

"Frances delves deeply into the history of mental illness, makes his arguments crisply, and has good personal stories to tell. He's articulate and learned. . . . He's in favor of not medicating, and thus muffling, all the offbeat pain and beauty out of existence."
—Dwight Garner, *New York Times*

"The man knows what he's talking about. . . . Frances has refined and critiqued, like no other, the new mental ailments of the diagnostic manual."   —*Der Spiegel*

"Authoritative. . . . Valuable. . . . This is a detailed, nicely constructed account by a highly qualified and well-connected psychiatrist with intimate knowledge of the process. The book is clearly written and surprisingly easy reading."
—The Royal Australian and New Zealand College of Psychiatrists

"Empirically grounded, learned, and engrossing—this is a godsend for the history of medicine."   —*Süddeutsche Zeitung*

"Professional and intelligible. . . . A fundamental book on the past, present, and future of psychiatric diagnoses and an impressive plea for the right to be normal."   —*Berliner Zeitung*

"*Saving Normal* is a clear, convincing, and essential discussion of the twin epidemics facing modern psychiatry: undertreatment of the truly ill and overtreatment of the basically well. It holds immense potential to improve patients' lives."   —Josh Bazell, M.D., *New York Times* bestselling author of *Beat the Reaper: A Novel*

"A passionate, intelligently written defense of human normality. This book deserves attention far beyond America."   —*Die Zeit*

"With his effort to 'save normality,' Frances hits the mark. . . . A book that should gain influence and the broadest possible reach. . . . Frances is an eloquent and sharp-tongued critic."   —*Die Presse*

"An indispensable guide for professional and lay readers."
—*Library Journal*

SAVING NORMAL

An Insider's Revolt Against Out-of-Control Psychiatric Diagnosis, DSM-5, Big Pharma, and the Medicalization of Ordinary Life

ALLEN FRANCES, M.D.

WILLIAM MORROW
An Imprint of HarperCollinsPublishers

A hardcover edition of this book was published in 2013 by William Morrow, an imprint of HarperCollins Publishers.

FIRST WILLIAM MORROW PAPERBACK EDITION PUBLISHED 2014.

Designed by Jamie Lynn Kerner

Library of Congress Cataloging-in-Publication Data has been applied for.

ISBN 978-0-06-222926-7

14 15 16 17 18 OV/RRD 10 9 8 7 6 5 4 3 2 1

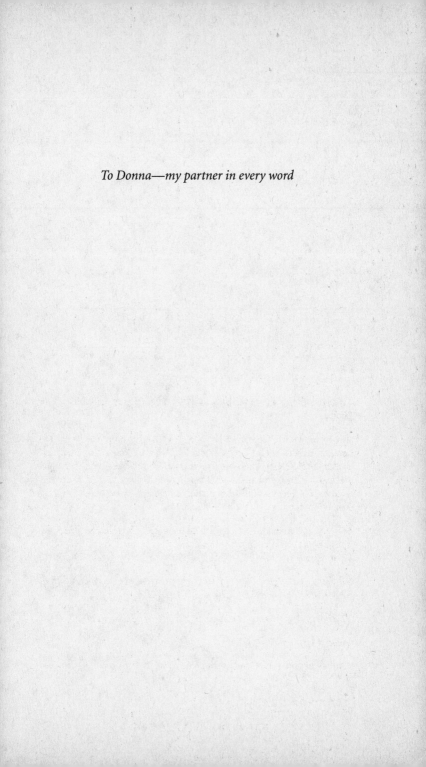

To Donna—my partner in every word

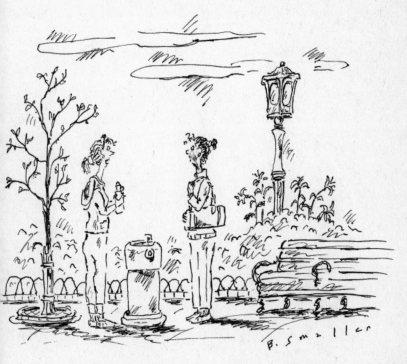

"*Evan has a syndrome where he cheats on me and does a lot of recreational drugs, but I forget the medical name for it.*"

CONTENTS

PREFACE

*I can calculate the movement of stars but
not the madness of men.*
ISAAC NEWTON

SOMETIMES YOU CAN get into a whole lot of trouble just minding your own business at a cocktail party. The time was May 2009. The party was a gathering of psychiatrists attending the annual meeting of the American Psychiatric Association. The place was the Asian Art Museum in San Francisco. The trouble was getting stuck in a bitter, public controversy about the nature of "normal" and the proper role of psychiatry in defining it.

I happened to be in town for something else and really had no interest in the meetings, but the party was a nice chance to catch up with old friends. For almost a decade, I had been pretty much a dropout from psychiatry—retiring early to care for my ailing wife, to babysit my mob of grandkids, to read, and to be a beach bum. Previously, my work life had been driven, probably qualifying as hyperactive. I led the Task Force that developed *DSM-IV* and also chaired the department of psychiatry at Duke, treated many patients, did research, and wrote some books and papers. It seemed like I was always chasing the clock and losing the race. Even a furtive look at the sports section of the *New York Times* felt like a stolen and forbidden pleasure. It was now a delight to simply kick back, read Thucydides, feel the sun on my face and the wind in what was left of my hair. No e-mail address, few phone calls, and absolutely no responsibilities beyond my family.

I have only one superstition—an irrational, but abiding, belief in the law of averages, that things equal out in the end. I know they don't—but superstitions die hard. I think the probability gods were bored the night of the party and decided to use me for their entertainment. Perhaps they had calculated that my life had become too carefree. Why not even the score by throwing my way a few chance tranquility-disrupting conversations? Within an hour, my comfortable sideline perch was lost, and I was forced to take sides in what has become a civil war for the heart of psychiatry—fighting a mostly losing battle to protect normality from medicalization and psychiatry from overexpansion.

Why me and why that night? It happens that several of my friends were bubbling over with excitement about their leading roles in preparing *DSM-5*. They could talk of little else. *DSM* stands for *Diagnostic and Statistical Manual*. Until 1980, *DSMs* were deservedly obscure little books that no one much cared about or read. Then *DSM-III* burst on the scene—a very fat book that quickly became a cultural icon, a perennial best seller, and the object of undue worship as the "bible" of psychiatry. Because it sets the crucial boundary between normality and mental illness, *DSM* has gained a huge societal significance and determines all sorts of important things that have an enormous impact on people's lives—like who is considered well and who is sick; what treatment is offered; who pays for it; who gets disability benefits; who is eligible for mental health, school, vocational, and other services; who gets to be hired for a job, can adopt a child, or pilot a plane, or qualifies for life insurance; whether a murderer is a criminal or a mental patient; what should be the damages awarded in lawsuits; and much, much more.

Having worked for twenty years on the periodically updated editions of the *DSM* (including *DSM-III*, *DSM-IIIR*, and *DSM-IV*), I knew the pitfalls and was wary about the risks inherent in any revision. In contrast, my friends were new to the game and excited about their role in preparing *DSM-5*. They intended to add many new mental disorders and to loosen the rules on how to diagnose the existing ones—they were overvaluing hoped-for benefits, blind to the downsides.

I understood their enthusiasm and eagerness to make a difference. Back in 1987, a week after finding out I would lead the *DSM-IV* effort, I took a long walk on the beach. I am not usually a person given to brooding, but I had much to think about. For about an hour, I felt an exhilarating sense of power as I plotted possible ways to change and improve psychiatry. My concern was that psychiatric diagnosis had come too far, too fast, and was changing too rapidly—there were too many categories and too many people being diagnosed. My three bright ideas were to raise the bar for disorders that seemed too easy to diagnose, to collapse together or eliminate the disorders that didn't make much sense, and to describe personality by flexible numbers, not rigid names.

In the second hour, reality set in and forced me to shoot down every one of my own pet projects. On reflection, I realized that in trying to correct problems I'd be creating new ones. And, more to the point, I realized that there was no reason why I (or anyone else) should trust me or my pet ideas. All changes to the diagnostic system should be science driven and evidenced based, not influenced by my personal whims or anyone else's. The method for doing *DSM-IV* needed to emphasize checks and balances in order to protect against individuality, arbitrariness, and diagnostic creativity. We would require that new proposals be subjected to a probing review of the scientific literature meant to focus on its risks and pitfalls. There would be painstaking data reanalyses and field trials. We would deep-six everything risky and/or without clear scientific merit. My hunch that high standards would eliminate almost all changes turned out to be true—there weren't compelling scientific data to back up the many proposals we eventually received. The basic science of psychiatry was daily coming up with exciting insights into how the brain works, but none of this translated one bit into how we should diagnose and treat patients.

I knew that we couldn't afford mistakes in *DSM-IV*, even small ones. *DSM* had become too powerful for its own good and for society's. Even seemingly minor changes could have a disastrous impact. And now *DSM-5* seemed poised to make some really big errors. In aggregate, the new disorders promoted so blithely by my friends would create tens of millions of new "patients." I pictured all these normal-enough people being captured in *DSM-5*'s excessively wide diagnostic net, and I worried that many would be exposed to unnecessary medicine with possibly dangerous side effects. The drug companies would be licking their chops figuring out how best to exploit the inviting new targets for their well-practiced disease mongering.

I was keenly alive to the risks because of painful firsthand experience—despite our efforts to tame excessive diagnostic exuberance, *DSM-IV* had since been misused to blow up the diagnostic bubble. Even though we had been boringly modest in our goals, obsessively meticulous in our methods, and rigidly conservative in our product, we failed to predict or prevent three new false epidemics of mental disorder in children—autism, attention deficit, and childhood bipolar disorder. And we did nothing to contain the rampant diagnostic inflation that was already expanding the boundary of psychiatry far beyond its competence. If a cautious and generally well-done *DSM-IV* had probably resulted in more harm than good, what were the likely negative effects of a carelessly done *DSM-5*, driven by its grand but quixotic ambition to be "paradigm shifting"?

The stakes were too high for me to ignore—both for the mislabeled new "patients" and for our society. Because of diagnostic inflation, an excessive proportion of people have come to rely on antidepressants, antipsychotics, antianxiety agents, sleeping pills, and pain meds. We are becoming a society of pill poppers. One out of every five U.S. adults uses at least one drug for a psychiatric problem; 11 percent of all adults took an antidepressant in 2010;[1] nearly 4 percent of our children are on a stimulant[2] and 4 percent of our teenagers are taking an antidepressant;[3] 25 percent of nursing home residents are given antipsychotics.[4] In Canada between 2005 and 2009, the use of psychostimulants went up by 36 percent, and SSRIs by 44 percent.[5]

Loose diagnosis is causing a national drug overdose of medication. Six percent of our people are addicted to prescription drugs, and there are now more emergency room visits and deaths due to legal prescription drugs than to illegal street drugs.[6] When their products are used carelessly, the drug companies can be as dangerous as the drug cartels. A case in point: Since 2005 there has been a remarkable eightfold increase in psychiatric prescriptions among our active duty troops. An incredible 110,000 soldiers are now taking at least one psychotropic drug, many are on more than one, and hundreds die every year from accidental overdoses.[7]

Psychiatric meds are now the star revenue producers for the drug companies—in 2011, over $18 billion for antipsychotics (an amazing 6 percent of all drug sales); $11 billion on antidepressants, and nearly $8 billion for ADHD drugs.[8] Expenditure on antipsychotics has tripled,[9] and antidepressant use nearly quadrupled from 1988 to 2008.[10] And the wrong doctors are giving out the pills. Eighty percent of prescriptions are written by primary-care physicians with little training in their proper use, under intense pressure from drug salespeople and misled patients, after rushed seven-minute appointments, with no systematic auditing.[11]

There is also a topsy-turvy misallocation of resources: way too much treatment is given to the normal "worried well" who are harmed by it; far too little help is available for those who are really ill and desperately need it. Two thirds of people with severe depression don't get treated for it, and many suffering with schizophrenia wind up in prisons. The writing is on the wall. "Normal" badly needs saving; sick people desperately require treatment. But *DSM-5* seemed to be moving in just the wrong direction, adding new diagnoses that would turn everyday anxiety, eccentricity, forgetting, and bad eating habits into mental disorders. Meanwhile the truly ill would be even more ignored as psychiatry expanded its boundaries to include many who are better considered normal.

They say the road to hell is paved with good intentions and bad unintended consequences. I was shocked by the naïve enthusiasm of the people working on *DSM-5*. Where they saw golden opportunities, I saw grave risks. Diagnostic exuberance can be bad for our health—as individuals and as a society.

By far the most disturbing conversation was with one of my oldest friends in psychiatry—a man of wisdom, experience, and integrity whose entire career had been dedicated to reducing the suffering caused by schizophrenia. He was convinced that *DSM-5* could make a game-changing difference by introducing a new diagnosis called "psychosis risk syndrome" that would encourage the early identification and preventive treatment of youngsters who might otherwise eventually become schizophrenic. My friend wanted to provide an ounce of early prevention that could substitute for a pound of later cure. Once the brain has already become sick, it is harder to make it well again— the more practiced are the circuits generating delusions and hallucination, the more difficult it will eventually be to turn them off. How wonderful then to prevent schizophrenia altogether, or failing that, at least to reduce the overall burden of the illness.

My friend's goal was noble, but there were five compelling strikes against it. Strike 1: most people getting the scary-sounding diagnosis "psychosis risk" would in fact be mislabeled—in the normal course of events, only a very small proportion would ever become psychotic. Strike 2: there is no proven way to prevent psychosis, even in those really at risk for developing it. Strike 3: many people would suffer collateral damage—receiving unnecessary antipsychotic drugs that can cause obesity, diabetes, heart disease, and likely a shortened life expectancy. Strike 4: think of the stigma and worry caused by the completely misleading implication that psychosis is just around the corner. Strike 5: since when is having a "risk" the same as having a "disease"? I tried but failed to change his mind, or even to open it the slightest bit. "Psychosis risk" was off and running. My friend's dream would surely cause a nightmare of disastrous unintended consequences.

As I drifted around the party, I met many other friends working on *DSM-5* who were similarly excited by their pet innovations and soon discovered that I personally qualified for many of the new disorders that were being suggested by them for inclusion for *DSM-5*. My gorging on the delectable shrimp and ribs was *DSM-5* "binge eating disorder." My forgetting names and faces would be covered by *DSM-5* "minor neurocognitive disorder." My worries and sadness were going to be "mixed anxiety/depressive disorder." The grief I felt when my wife died was "major depressive disorder." My well-known hyperactivity and distractibility were clear signs of "adult attention deficit disorder." An hour of amiable chatting with old friends, and I had already acquired five new *DSM* diagnoses. And let's not forget my six-year-old identical twin grandsons—their temper tantrums were no longer just annoying; they had "temper dysregulation disorder."

Clearly *DSM-5* would make a mess. What to do? I had previously declined several requests to have a say. Bob Spitzer, the great psychiatric innovator who had been most responsible for creating *DSM-III*, had for years been sounding loud public alarms. He was upset that the American Psychiatric Association was forcing the people working on *DSM-5* to sign confidentiality agreements intended to protect APA's "intellectual property." Publishing profit should never trump the transparency needed to produce a safe and quality *DSM*. Bob was dead right, and I knew it. He had often asked for my support in his efforts to help get *DSM-5* on the right track, but to my shame, I had repeatedly refused to speak up. My lifelong inclination has always been to steer clear of controversy, and this one promised to be particularly unappealing. I also felt it was bad form to comment on the work of my successors, and besides, I knew Bob to be a good and tireless fighter who could more than hold his own in public debate.

But the disturbing conversations at the party finally shook my complacency and forced me into the fray. It was not just a matter of *DSM-5* having a closed and secretive process; it would likely produce a very dangerous product. If "psychosis risk" made it into *DSM-5*, innocent kids might become obese and die early receiving unnecessary medication for a fake diagnosis. *DSM-5* was going to create public-health problems, and the public needed to have a say. I realized it would be selfish and cowardly to cop out with the excuse that Bob alone could do all the heavy lifting. I would have to risk friendships, break ranks with organized psychiatry, and come off my beloved beach. Janet Williams, Bob's wife and closest collaborator on *DSM-III*, also happened to be at the party. I walked over and told her that Bob could count me in. *DSM-5* was too important to be left in the hands of a group of well-meaning, but badly misguided, "experts."

It is now four years later. I have spoken to the APA leadership; written four warning letters to the APA Trustees; posted countless blogs; published numerous editorials and papers; given talks at professional and public meetings and appeared on radio and television—all warning about the risks that *DSM-5* will mislabel normal people, promote diagnostic inflation, and encourage inappropriate medication use. I have not been alone in trying to save normal. Many other individuals, mental health organizations, professional journals, and the press have loudly sounded the very same alarm. We have had some positive impact—at the eleventh hour, *DSM-5* dropped some of its most dangerous proposals. But overall we failed. *DSM-5* pushes psychiatric diagnosis in the wrong direction, will create new false epidemics, and promotes even more medication misuse. The right goal for *DSM-5* would have been diagnostic restraint and deflation, not a further unwarranted expansion of diagnosis and treatment.

This book is my reaction to the excesses—part mea culpa, part j'accuse, part cri de coeur. It provides an insider's despairing view of what has gone wrong and also offers a practical road map back to a safe and sane psychiatry. My goal is not only to help "save normal," but also to help save psychiatry. Psychiatry is a noble and essential profession, sound at its core, and extremely effective when done well. Our outcomes match or exceed what is achieved by most other medical specialties.[12] And being a mental health caregiver is a special privilege—we get to know our patients intimately, console their sorrows, and find ways to help them help themselves. We can cure many, help most, and provide compassion and advice for all. But psychiatry must stay within its proper competence and stick to what it does best—helping people who really need and can most benefit from our efforts. We should not be making patients of people who are basically normal and ignoring those who are really sick.

Psychiatry is certainly not alone in its overreaching—we are just a special case of the bloat and waste that characterize all of U.S. medicine. Commercial interests have hijacked the medical enterprise, putting profit before patients and creating a feeding frenzy of overdiagnosis, overtesting, and overtreatment. We spend twice as much on health care as other countries and have only mediocre outcomes to show for it. Some of our citizens are harmed by too much medical care, others by shameful neglect. Medicine and psychiatry both stand greatly in need of taming, pruning, reformulation, and redirection.

Real psychiatric disorders require prompt diagnosis and active treatment—they don't get better by themselves and become harder to treat the longer they are allowed to persist. In contrast, the unavoidable everyday problems of life are best resolved through our natural resilience and the healing powers of time. We are a tough species, the successful survivors of ten thousand generations of resourceful ancestors who had to make their precarious daily living and avoid ever-present dangers far beyond our coddled imagining. Our brains and our social structures are adapted to deal with the toughest of circumstances—we are fully capable of finding solutions to most of life's troubles without medical meddling, which often muddles the situation and makes it worse. As we drift ever more toward the wholesale medicalization of normality, we lose touch with our strong self-healing capacities—forgetting that most problems are not sickness and that only rarely is popping a pill the best solution.

But writing this book has a serious risk that I wouldn't have assumed were the risks of not writing it even greater. My nightmare scenario is that some people will do a selective reading and draw the completely incorrect and unintended conclusion that I am against psychiatric diagnosis and treatment. They may be overly influenced by my criticisms of the field when it is practiced poorly and miss my very strong endorsements of psychiatry when it is practiced well. My *DSM-IV* experience taught me that any word that can possibly be misused or misunderstood likely will be and that authors have to worry about the consequences that can follow not only from the proper use of their writings but also those that can result from the predictable distortions. I am already widely and misleadingly quoted by scientologists and other groups that are rabidly opposed to psychiatry. This book can be similarly misused by them to discourage people who desperately need help from getting it. Let us suppose this hypothetical chain of events—a basic misunderstanding of my message induces some people who need medicine to precipitously stop it, causing a relapse into illness that is accompanied by suicidal or violent behavior. Although not directly responsible, I would still have good reason to feel terrible.

Despite these realistic concerns, I decided to go ahead and write the book because the current massive overuse of psychotropic drugs in our country presents a much greater and more immediate danger. My hope is to simultaneously serve two purposes—first to alert people who don't need treatment to avoid it, but equally to encourage those who do need treatment to seek it out and to stick with it. My critique is directed only against the excesses of psychiatry, not its heart or soul. "Saving normal" and "saving psychiatry" are really two sides of the very same coin. Psychiatry needs to be saved from rushing in where it should fear to tread. Normal needs to be saved from the powerful forces trying to convince us that we are all sick.

PART I

Normality Under Siege

CHAPTER 1

What's Normal and What's Not?

The pool of normality is shrinking into a mere puddle.
Til Wykes

Before we begin saving normal, we need to figure out what it is. You might expect *normal* to be an approachable sort of word, confident in its popularity, safe in its preponderance over *abnormal*. Defining *normal* should be easy, and being normal should be a modest ambition. Not so. Normal has been badly besieged and is already sadly diminished. Dictionaries can't provide a satisfying definition; philosophers argue over its meaning; statisticians and psychologists measure it endlessly but fail to capture its essence; sociologists doubt its universality; psychoanalysts doubt its existence; and doctors of the mind and body are busily nipping away at its borders. Normal is losing all purchase—if only we look hard enough perhaps everyone will eventually turn out to be more or less sick. My task in this book will be to try to stop this steady, inexorable encroachment—to help save normal.

How Does the Dictionary Define Normal?

The word *normal* plays in many different arenas. It started its life in Latin as a carpenter's square and is still used in geometry to describe right angles and perpendiculars. Not surprisingly, normal then took on any number of right-minded connotations denoting the regular, standard, usual, routine, typical, average, run-of-the-mill, expected, habitual, universal, common, conforming, conventional, correct, or customary. From this, a short jump had normal describing good biological and psychological functioning—not physically sick, not mentally sick.[1]

The dictionary definitions of *normal* are all entirely and beguilingly tautological. To know what is normal you have to know what is abnormal. And guess how *abnormal* is defined in the dictionaries—those things that are not normal or regular or natural or typical or usual or conforming to a norm. Talk about circular tail chasing—each term is defined exclusively as the negative of the other; there is no real definition of either, and no meaningful definitional line between them.

The dichotomous terms "normal" and "abnormal" inspire a sense of familiar recognition and false familiarity. We instinctively intuit what they mean in a general way but find it inherently hard to pin them down when it gets to the specific. There is no universal and transcendental definition that works operationally to solve real-world sorting problems.

What Does Philosophy Say?

Surprisingly little. Philosophy has exerted itself endlessly to understand the deeper meanings of big concepts like reality and illusion, how we know things, the nature of human nature, truth, morality, justice, duty, love, beauty, greatness, goodness, evil, mortality, immortality, natural law, and on and on. Normal generally got lost in the philosophical shuffle—perhaps too ordinary and uninteresting to warrant deep philosophical thought.

This neglect finally ended with the Enlightenment attempt to apply philosophy to the more mundane problems of day-to-day living. Utilitarianism provided the first, and remains the only practical, philosophic guidance on how and where to set a boundary between "normal" and "mental disorder." The guiding assumptions are that "normal" has no universal meaning and can never be defined with precision by the spinning wheels of philosophical deduction—it is very much in the eye of the beholder and is changeable over time, place, and cultures. From this it follows that the boundary separating "normal" from "mental disorder" should be based not on abstract reasoning, but rather on the balance between the positive and the negative consequences that accrue from different choices. Always seek the "greatest good for the greatest number."[2] Make decisions depending on what measurably works best.

But there are also undeniable uncertainties in being a practical utilitarian, and even worse there are dangerous value land mines. "The greatest good for the greatest number" sounds great on paper, but how do you measure the quantities and how do you decide what's the good? It is no accident that utilitarianism is currently least popular in Germany, where Hitler gave it such an enduringly bad name. During World War II, it was statistically normal for the German population to act in barbaric ways that would be deemed decidedly abnormal before or since—all justified at the time on utilitarian grounds as necessary to provide for the greatest good of the master race. Statistical "normal" (based on the frequency of what is) temporarily badly trumped injunctive "normal" (the world as it should be or customarily had been).

Granted that, in the wrong hands, utilitarianism can be blind to good values and twisted by bad ones, it still remains the best or only philosophical guide when we embark on the difficult task of setting boundaries between the mentally "normal" and the mentally "abnormal." This is the approach we used in *DSM-IV*.

Can Statistics Dictate Normal?

Having previously befuddled linguistics and philosophy, normal next defeated statistics. This may be surprising. Statistics would seem perfectly poised to define normal by switching the method of analysis from playing with words to playing with numbers. The answer could come from the beautifully symmetrical shape of a normal bell curve. Whenever you measure things, there is never one absolutely perfect and replicable right answer. There is always a greater or lesser error of measurement that prevents us from reproducing the same answer every time—no matter how carefully we try and how wonderful is our measuring rod. It is inherently impossible for us to pin down the nature of anything with absolute precision. But a truly remarkable thing happens if we go to the trouble of taking enough measurements. Even though no one reading is perfectly accurate or predictable, the aggregate of all readings sort in the most perfectly predictable and the loveliest of curves. At the curve's peak is the most popular measure; then the successively less likely ones trail down on both sides as we move away from this golden mean.

The bell curve explains a great deal about how life works—most things about nature and about people follow its shape and deviate predictably around the mean. The distributions of every conceivable characteristic in the universe have been measured in enormous and painstakingly collected data sets. Miraculously, the same wonderful "normal curve" always emerges from what might otherwise appear to be a jumble of numbers. The curve provides remarkably precise predictive power on virtually everything that matters to our species and to the world.

Human beings are diverse in every one of our physical, emotional, intellectual, attitudinal, and behavioral characteristics, but our diversity is not at all random. We are "normally" distributed on a bell-shaped curve on any given trait that is continuously distributed in our population. IQ, height, weight, personality traits all cluster around a golden mean with the outliers sorting symmetrically on both sides.

The best way of summarizing this economically and systematically is the standard deviation (SD)—a technical term used in statistics to describe the way measures arrange themselves with reliable regularity around the mean. Being within one SD of the mean for height (which is 5′10″ for men in the United States with an SD of three inches) puts you in very popular territory joined by 68 percent of the population—34 percent will be just somewhat taller than the completely average guy (up to 6′1″) and 34 percent will be somewhat shorter (down to 5′7″). As you get much taller or much shorter you become more and more the rare bird—it gets lonelier and lonelier out there on either side of the further reaches of the bell curve. Only 5 percent of the population drifts off by more than two SDs —in this remote region we have the 2.5 percent of really tall men (over 6′4″) and the 2.5 percent of short men (under 5′4″). This is the region of the bell curve at the extreme right and the extreme left, far away from the popular golden mean. Suppose we take it even further and go out to three SDs—here we are in the really rarefied territory with the very few men who are over 6′7″or under 5′1″.[3]

This brings us to the question of the moment—can we use statistics in some simple and precise way to define mental normality? Can the bell curve provide a scientific guide in deciding who is mentally normal and who is not? Conceptually, the answer is "why not," but practically the answer is "hell no." In theory, we could arbitrarily decide that the most troubled among us (5 percent, or 10 percent, or 30 percent or whatever) would be defined as mentally ill and that the rest of us are normal. Then we could develop survey instruments, score everyone, draw up the curves, set the boundary line, and thus label the sick. But in practice it just doesn't work that way. There are just too many statistical, contextual, and value judgments that perplex a simple statistical solution.

First, people on the immediate opposite sides of whatever boundary is set will look almost exactly alike—how silly to call one sick, the other healthy. People who are 6′3″ and 6′4″ are both tall. And what percentage to choose? If there are just a few mental health clinicians in a developing country, only the most severely disturbed will appear mentally disordered—so perhaps the boundary will be set so that only 1 percent are not normal. In a New York City saturated with therapists, the level required for disorder is radically defined down and perhaps the boundary would be set at 30 percent or more. It gets completely arbitrary and the pretty curve has no way of telling us where to draw the line.

We must reconcile to there not being any simple standard to decide the question of how many of us are abnormal. The normal curve tells us a great deal about the distribution of everything from quarks to koalas, but it doesn't dictate to us where normal ends and abnormal begins. A ranting psychotic is far enough away from mean to be recognized as mentally sick by your aunt Tilly, but how do you decide when everyday anxiety or sadness is severe enough to be considered mental disorder? One thing does seem perfectly clear. On the statistical face of it, it is ridiculous to stretch disorder so elastically that the near average person can qualify. Shouldn't most people be normal?

What Does the Doctor Say About Normal?

Until the late 1800s, medicine was ruled by the dogma that health and illness were determined by the relative quantities of the four bodily humors—blood, phlegm, and yellow and black bile. This seems quaint and daffy now, but it was one of mankind's most enduring ideas (outlasting by far the dogma that the sun revolves around the Earth). Humoral theory was the commonly held belief of a hundred generations of the smartest people in the world and governed medical practice for four millennia. The ticket to normality was achieving perfect balance and harmony of the bodily fluids—nothing in excess, nothing lacking. Only in the late nineteenth century did dramatic advances in physiology, pathology, and neuroscience finally relegate humoral theory to the dusty closet of atavistic medical curiosities.[4]

But, despite all of its acknowledged wonders, modern medical science has never provided a workable definition of "health" or "illness"—in either the physical or the mental realms. Many have tried and all have failed. Take, for example, the World Health Organization's definition[5]: "Health is a state of complete physical, mental, and social well-being and not merely the absence of infirmity." Who among us would dare claim health if it requires meeting this impossibly high standard? Health loses value as a concept when it is so unobtainable that everyone is at least partly sick. The definition also exudes culture and context-sensitive value judgments. Who gets to define what is "complete" physical, mental, and social well-being? Is someone sick because his body aches from hard work or he feels sad after a disappointment or is in a family feud? And are the poor inherently sicker because they have fewer resources to achieve the complete well-being required of "health"?

More realistic modern definitions of health focus not on the perfectibility of life, but on the lack of definable disease. This is better, but there is no bright-line definition of physical disease and certainly nothing that works across time, place, and culture. How do we decide what is normal in continuum situations like blood pressure, or cholesterol, or blood sugar, or bone density? Is a slow-growing prostate cancer in an old person best diagnosed and treated aggressively as disease—or left alone because neglect may be much less dangerous than treatment? Is the average expectable forgetting that occurs in old age the disease of dementia or the unavoidable degenerative destiny of a brain grown old? Is a very short child just short or in need of hormone injections?[6]

Why No Lab Tests to Define Normal in Psychiatry

The human brain is by far the most complicated thing in the known universe. The brain has 100 billion neurons, each of which is connected to 1,000 other neurons—making for a grand total of 100 trillion synaptic connections. Every second, an average of 1,000 signals cross each of these synapses; each signal is modulated by 1,500 proteins and mediated by one or more of dozens of neurotransmitters.[7] Brain development is even more improbable—a miracle of intricately choreographed sequential nerve cell migration. Each nerve has to somehow find just its right spot and make just the right connections. Given all the many steps involved and all the possible things that can go wrong, you might want to place your bet on Murphy's Law and chaos theory—the odds seem to be stacked against normal brain functioning. The weird and wonderful thing is that we work as well as we do—the improbable result of exquisitely wrought DNA engineering that has to accomplish trillions and trillions of steps. But any supercomplicated system will have its occasional chaotic glitches. Things can and do go wrong in many different ways to produce each disease, which makes it hard for medical science to take giant steps.

The two most exciting advances in the entire history of biology are unraveling the workings of the human brain and breaking the genetic code. No one could have predicted that we would have come so far and so fast. But there has also been a great disappointment. Although we have learned a great deal about brain functioning, we have not yet figured out ways of translating basic science into clinical psychiatry. The powerful new tools of molecular biology, genetics, and imaging have not yet led to laboratory tests for dementia or depression or schizophrenia or bipolar or obsessive-compulsive disorder or for any other mental disorders. The expectation that there would be a simple gene or neurotransmitter or circuitry explanation for any mental disorder has turned out to be naive and illusory.

We still do not have a single laboratory test in psychiatry. Because there is always more variability in the results within the mental disorder category than between it and normal or other mental disorders, none of the promising biological findings has ever qualified as a diagnostic test. The brain has provided us no low-hanging fruit—thousands of studies on hundreds of putative biological markers have so far come up empty. Why the gaping disconnect—so much knowledge and so little practical utility? As Roger Sperry put it in his Nobel Prize in Medicine acceptance speech: "The more we learn, the more we recognize the unique complexity of any one individual intellect, the stronger the conclusion becomes that the individuality inherent in our brain networks makes that of fingerprints or facial features gross and simple by comparison."[8] Teasing out the heterogeneous underlying mechanisms of mental disorder will be the work of lifetimes. There will not be one pathway to schizophrenia; there may be dozens, perhaps hundreds or thousands.

The brain reveals its secrets only slowly and in very small packages. Every exciting finding turns out to be a tease—providing no simple answers, rarely replicating fully in the next study, uncovering more heterogeneous complexity than it explains. To use a baseball analogy—there are no grand slams in this work and no walks, just plenty of strikeouts and at best the occasional single. And this will be a very slow and retail slog, not any one great leap forward. We will not have biological markers to set the boundary between normal and mental disorder until we understand the multitudinous mechanisms causing the different forms of psychopathology. And there won't be a Newton or an Einstein or a Darwin to provide a grand unifying biological theory of normality and mental disorder—just patient scientists each working for decades to elucidate one very tiny piece of an enormous, trillion-piece jigsaw puzzle. Causes for mental disorder, as they are discovered, will (as with breast cancer) explain only a small percentage of the cases. The first real step in this advance will be laboratory tests for Alzheimer's dementia, probably ready to come online sometime in the next few years.

The absence of biological tests is a huge disadvantage for psychiatry. It means that all of our diagnoses are now based on subjective judgments that are inherently fallible and prey to capricious change. It is like having to diagnose pneumonia without having any tests for the viruses or bacteria that cause the various types of lung infection.

Can Psychology Ride to the Rescue?

Sadly no. We can do psychological tests on people till they are bleary-eyed and blue in the face and still not be much further along in setting the boundary between who is normal and who is not. The limitation of almost all tests used by psychologists is that the distribution of their results follows our old friend—the bell-shaped normal curve. The test can tell us with remarkable precision just where a given person stands with respect to his comparison group, and knowing someone's standard deviation position relative to the mean often has considerable predictive value. But the testing doesn't tell us where to set the cutoffs for what is normal. That is determined by context, not by test score.

Take IQ testing. Two standard deviations below the mean of 100 put you at 70 and predicts the likelihood of school and life difficulties. Two standard deviations above normal put you at 130 and predicts academic and career success. But there isn't any reason to think that having a IQ of 70 is really different from having one of 71 or even 75.[9] There is a 5-point error of measurement in the test, many factors may have interfered with optimal test taking, and some people perform in life much better or worse than you might expect just from their IQ.

Selecting 70 as the unique cutoff for clearly disordered intellectual ability is purely an arbitrary convenience that has no particular significance other than that it selects for the lowest 2.5 percent of the population. These individuals are likely to qualify for special services and dispensations that are denied their near and almost identical neighbors. But there is nothing sacred about the two standard deviations below 100 cutoff at IQ 70—it doesn't have a real world meaning. Slightly higher or slightly lower cutoffs would make equal or more sense, depending on the situation. If more resources are available, services should be offered to those with higher IQs than 70. In some environments, people with an IQ of 70 do just fine. And who says that two standard deviations should be the cutoff? Why not one or three or one and a half? The choice is always arbitrary and driven by context, not statistics.

This gets lost in translation. A recent galling example followed the Supreme Court ruling that it is unconstitutional to execute anyone who is suffering from mental retardation. Life versus death now depends on the silly, artificial nondistinction of having an IQ of 70, rather than 71.[10]

What would happen if we applied the two SD cutoff (2.5 percent) to psychiatry and suddenly required that people be that far removed from the golden mean of mental health before they could merit a diagnosis of mental disorder. Psychiatrists and other mental health workers would mostly be put out of business and have to collect unemployment insurance. One hundred years ago, psychiatry was limited to the very severely ill housed in hospitals, and very few people were employed caring for them. We have since worked our way up the bell curve much closer to the mean—so that 20 to 25 percent are currently considered mentally disordered, and we have more than half a million people caring for them. Using the psychological test paradigm, we can compare people very precisely to one another but have no way to decide whether to draw the line between normal and abnormal at 2.5 percent or 25 percent of the population.

Do Sociologists or Anthropologists Have the Answer?

Nope, again. Human customs around the world vary too dramatically across time, place, and cultures for there to be any ready answer to what is normal across all of them. Contrast the million or so people willing to starve to death during the siege of Leningrad (rather than break the norm against eating the readily available protein from human flesh) with a perfectly normal New Guinean who until fairly recently wouldn't think twice about cooking up the body or eating the brains of his lately departed enemy. Two hundred years ago, the normal age of marriage everywhere in the world was around puberty (and it still is in some places), but this is now deemed criminal in our society. With longer life expectancies, it is normal now to marry at an age that only recently would be when we could reasonably expect to be dead.

Cultural universals are the exception, with just a few rock-solid cultural norms (e.g., no murder within tribe, incest restrictions, some sort of family structure). Cultures differ dramatically in their conception of normal because they face different survival challenges. Geographically isolated Inuit avoided inbreeding by finding it normal to offer up the wife as bedmate to passing strangers. In contrast, classical Greeks and modern Arabs have elaborated the strongest of strictures preventing any sort of female exposure to strange genes so that the inheritance of property would surely follow patriarchal bloodlines. Aboriginals desperately needing protein find ants to be a perfectly normal food source—whereas habitually eating them in Los Angeles might qualify one for the *DSM* mental disorder known as pica. And context can be all—murder is heroic and normal when committed against threatening outsiders; it is heinous and abnormal within the tribe.

Even within a given time and place there are conflicting norms. Durkheim[11] fathered sociology more than a century ago with fascinating statistics documenting the predictable divergence between the morally normal and the statistically normal. Societies all prohibit crime, but crime abounds everywhere—perfectly normal from a statistical point of view, but perfectly abnormal from a legal one. Societies also tend to prohibit suicide, but the suicide rate in each country is remarkably consistent year after year, even though suicide is the most personal of human decisions. Ruthlessness may be prized both among gangbangers and corporate leaders, but it will take very different forms and be rewarded and punished in very different ways.

Inbuilt hard wiring also makes for different tendencies in gender norms. Males are more adapted to fight for love and glory—consonant with their existential struggle for access to females, their prominent role in war with other tribes, and the needs of the hunt. Females are more likely to have inborn skills in nurturing and in food gathering. But there are huge individual and cross-cultural differences and there is far from any fixed normal when it comes to male or female behavior.

So at least for now (until Facebook succeeds in homogenizing the planet into one vast, dull social network), normal is a sociological will-o'-the-wisp. There is no norm for normal.

What About Freud?

Freud was a very smart guy who was overrated when he was alive and pays the price now of being greatly underrated. His insights on how the mind works were somewhat hit or miss, but he certainly hit a home run in his appreciation of the powerful role of inborn, unconscious instinct in guiding the most exalted and also the most mundane of everyday behaviors. Freud delighted in uncovering the underlying similarities in dreams, works of art, myths, and in the neurotic and psychotic symptoms of psychiatric patients. He used dreams to uncover the meaning of symptoms, symptoms to uncover the meaning of myths, and his patients' fantasies to interpret Hamlet and Oedipus. Literature and myth could be used to explain his patients, and his patients' illnesses reciprocally helped him to explain literature and myth.

The psychoanalytic model tended to be all-inclusive, but there was one notable exception—there is no real place in it for normal. Freud emphasized the ways we are all in the same boat. He saw no great qualitative difference between the artist and the lunatic, and both resemble the rest of us every night when we dream. We all must repress forbidden impulses, which are always at the ready to pop out in dreams, symptoms, or works of art—we are different only in the balance of forces and their means of expression. No one is ever completely normal for Freud; everyone is neurotic and could use more insight. The most any successful treatment can ever hope to achieve is to turn neurotic misery into everyday human unhappiness. There is no normal, no cutoff marker saying treatment is necessary, or when it should end.[12] The great unspoken paradox of the arduous process of psychoanalysis is that the best patients are the ones who never really needed it in the first place.

Abnormal Is Also Hard to Define

Proteus was the shape-shifting Greek sea god, a familiar of the Fates who knew the secrets of past, present, and future. But Proteus was wily and reluctant to share his knowledge—except if someone could grab him while he slept and hang on as he executed a succession of rapidly morphing, terrifying, and difficult-to-contain form changes. Not easy work holding a firm grip on a roaring lion that can suddenly transform itself into flowing water, or a charging bull, or anything else you can possibly imagine. Proteus is the personification of things that are liquid, elusive, indefinite, and mutable—things that defy clear definition.

"Mental disorder" and "normality" are both extremely protean concepts—each so amorphous, heterogeneous, and changeable in shape that we can never establish fixed boundaries between them. The definitions of mental disorder generally require the presence of distress, disability, dysfunction, dyscontrol, and/or disadvantage. This sounds better as alliteration than it works as operational guide. How much distress, disability, dysfunction, dyscontrol, and disadvantage must there be, and of what kind?[13] I have reviewed dozens of definitions of mental disorder (and have written one myself in *DSM-IV*) and find none of them the slightest bit helpful either in determining which conditions should be considered mental disorders and which not, or in deciding who is sick and who is not.[14-18]

Not having a useful definition of mental disorder creates a gaping hole at the center of psychiatric classification, resulting in two unanswered conundrums: how to decide which disorders to include in the diagnostic manual and how to decide whether a given individual has a mental disorder. Binge eating was once considered a sin; should it now be a psychiatric disorder? Is the forgetting of old age an illness or just old age? Is having sex with a teenager just a crime or also a sign of craziness? And in evaluating any given person, we lack a general definition of mental disorder to help us decide whether he is normal or a patient, mad or bad.[19, 20]

The mental disorders included in *DSM-5* have not gained their official status through any rational process of elimination. They made it into the system and have survived because of practical necessity, historical accident, gradual accretion, precedent, and inertia—not because they met some independent set of abstract and universal definitional criteria.[21, 22] No surprise then that the *DSM* disorders are something of a hodgepodge, not internally consistent or mutually exclusive. Some mental disorders describe short-term states, others lifelong personality; some reflect inner misery, others bad behavior; some represent problems rarely or never seen in normals, others are just slight accentuations of the everyday; some reflect too little self-control, others too much; some are intrinsic to the person, others are culturally determined; some begin early in infancy, others emerge only late in life; some affect thought, others emotions, behaviors, interpersonal relations; some seem more biological, others more psychological or social; some are supported by thousands of research studies, others by a mere handful; some may clearly belong in *DSM*, others could have been left out and perhaps should be eliminated; some are clearly defined, others not; and there are complex permutations of all of these possible differences.

I sometimes joke that the only way to define mental disorder is "that which clinicians treat; researchers research; educators teach; and insurance companies pay for." Unfortunately, this practical "definition" is elastic, tautological, and potentially self-serving—following practice habits rather than guiding them. The greater the number of mental health clinicians, the greater the number of life conditions that work their way into becoming disorders. Only six disorders were listed in the initial census of mental patients in the mid-nineteenth century; now there are close to two hundred. Society has a seemingly insatiable capacity (even hunger) to accept and endorse newly minted mental disorders that help to define and explain away its emerging concerns.

Are Mental Disorders Diseases, Myths, or Something Else?

Some radical critics of psychiatry have seized on its definitional ambiguities to argue that the profession should not exist at all. They take the difficulty in finding a clear definition of mental disorder as evidence that the concept has no useful meaning—if mental disorders are not anatomically defined medical diseases, they must be "myths," and there is no real need to bother diagnosing them. This position is most appealing to libertarians concerned with preserving patient freedom of choice from what they perceive to be the enslaving snares of psychiatry. "Saving normal" is taken by them to its logical extreme—the extremely illogical position that everyone is normal.

This shibboleth can be believed only by armchair theorists with no real life experience in having, living with, or treating mental illness. However difficult to define, psychiatric disorder is an all-too-painful reality for those who suffer from it and for those who care about them.[23] Saving normal, as I use the term, is not meant to deny the value of psychiatric diagnosis and treatment. Rather, it is an effort to keep psychiatry doing what it does well within its appropriate limits.

It is equally dangerous at either extreme—to have either an expanding concept of mental disorder that eliminates normal or to have an expanding concept of normal that eliminates mental disorder.

The best way to understand the essence of mental disorder—what it is and what it is not—is to compare the balls and strikes calls of three different umpires. Most of epistemology boils down to their competing opinions on how well we can ever apprehend reality.

Umpire One: "There are balls and there are strikes and I call them as they are."

Umpire Two: "There are balls and there are strikes and I call them as I see them."

Umpire Three: "There are no balls and there are no strikes until I call them."

Umpire One believes that mental disorders are real "diseases"; Umpire Three that they are fanciful "myths"; Umpire Two that they are something in between—useful constructs that provide no more (but no less) than a best current guess on how to sort psychiatric distress.

Umpire One has great faith in our ability to detect the true essence of things. For him, mental disorders will soon reveal their secrets through scientific study. This optimism was shared by most biological psychiatrists until about fifteen years ago but, except for a few diehards, is now rapidly fading away. Billions of research dollars have failed to produce convincing evidence that any mental disorder is a discrete disease entity with a unitary cause.[24, 25, 26] Dozens of different candidate genes have been "found," but in follow-up studies each turned out to be fool's gold. Mental disorders are too heterogeneous in presentation and in causality to be considered simple diseases; instead each of our currently defined disorders will eventually turn out to be many different diseases. For now at least, Umpire One has been called out on strikes.[27, 28, 29]

Umpire Three presents just the opposite view—the skeptical and solipsistic doubt that man can ever catch protean reality by the tail and know things as they truly are. He would argue that mental disorders are no more than arbitrary and sometimes noxious "myths" that unfairly restrict the freedom of choice of psychiatric patients. He worries about the slippery slope that eventually could be extended to other vulnerable groups.[30] Indeed, there is reason for this concern—psychiatric diagnosis is now being abused for preventive detention of rapists in the United States and peasants complaining about corruption in China and previously was an excuse to hospitalize political dissidents in the Soviet Union.

It is of course imperative that we protect against the misuse of psychiatry in the service of legal or political masters—but Umpire Three far overstates his case. Mental disorders are not myths. Though not a discrete "disease entity" (like, say, a brain tumor or a stroke), schizophrenia produces profound and prolonged "dis-ease"—that is, distress and incapacity. The patterns of its presentation are clearly recognizable, can be reliably diagnosed, run in families, have brain imaging correlates, predict course, and respond to specific treatments. Schizophrenia is real enough and no psychiatric invention for those who suffer from it and for their loved ones.

Umpire Two has the firmest grasp on elusive reality, paradoxically because he understands and accepts that we can know it only partially. Of course, reality is "protean"—constantly changing shape and hard to hold. No doubt there is an enormous gap between things as they really are and things as we perceive them—and not just in psychiatry. Only 4 percent of our known universe can be directly detected by our senses—the rest of its energy and matter remaining "dark" to us. The quantum world is so weirdly discordant with our own that even the physicists who can mathematically predict its every characteristic cannot find an intuitive way to relate to it. And how can light manage to be a wave that suddenly turns into a particle just when we choose to look at it a certain way.

Elusive reality does not discourage Umpire Two. We don't have to fully perceive or understand the underlying nature of our world to negotiate it well. Our senses and reasoning powers evolved as they did because they work just fine in the everyday, nonphilosophical business of survival. Mental constructs of reality are imperfect, but indispensable, ways to organize the otherwise bewildering phenomena of the world.

Umpire Two "calls them as he sees them." Mental disorders are not real diseases as Umpire One might wish; but neither are they the dangerous myths feared by Umpire Three. Instead he follows a down-to-earth brand of utilitarian pragmatism. His umpire's eye is fixed on what works best—not distracted by biological reductionism or rationalist doubt. He accepts that we are constantly constructing perceptions and finding temporary meanings that are useful, but never completely accurate. Our classification of mental disorders is no more than a collection of fallible and limited constructs that seeks but never finds the truth—but this remains our best current way of communicating about, treating, and researching mental disorders.

Schizophrenia is a useful construct—not myth, not disease. It is a description of a particular set of psychiatric problems, not an explanation of their cause. Someday we will have a much more accurate understanding and more precise ways of describing these same problems. But for now, schizophrenia is very valuable in our day-to-day work. And so are the other *DSM* disorders. It is good to know and use the *DSM* definitions, but not to reify or worship them.[31,32]

Defining Disorder Around the World

What about the potentially distorting lens of culture? Do mental disorders present the same way everywhere or does each culture need its own diagnostic system? The answer seems to be that one size usually fits almost all. Although "normal" behavior is variable across cultures, the specific mental disorders are pretty uniform. Dementia, psychosis, mania, depression, panic attacks, anxiety, obsessive-compulsive disorder, and the personality disorders have been described in all past

ages and in all places and are found today in epidemiological studies wherever in the world these are conducted. When rates of disorder
differ (e.g., blacks being diagnosed more often with schizophrenia in
the United States), it is because of bias or cultural blind spots in the
raters, not real differences in the patients they are rating.[33]

There are two diagnostic systems in current, overlapping use
around the world—*DSM-5* (soon to be translated into about twenty-
two languages) and ICD-10, developed by the World Health Organization (translated into forty-two languages).[34] *DSM-5* and ICD-10 are
really very similar; which is not surprising, since they are closely related sibs. Both are no more than minor modifications of the same
parent (*DSM-III*) and were prepared at the same time and with some
efforts to achieve harmony. As with sibs, there is a rivalry between systems. The *DSM*s have so far been more influential, but it will be several
years before we can judge whether *DSM-5* or ICD-11 (planned for publication around 2016) will win the next round of the competition. For
now, the relative merits of *DSM* and ICD are pretty obvious—*DSM* is
used much more often in research; they are about equal for clinical
work in the developed countries; and ICD works better when a simpler
system is needed in the developing world.[35]

The more fascinating question is why both diagnostic systems have
gained such universal applicability across all the races and cultures of
the world. Clearly we humans are more alike than we are different, resembling one another closely in the things that count toward defining
normal and mental disorder.

There are no genetically caused racial differences in mental disorder. How come there is such uniformity? Compared to other species, humans have a remarkably homogeneous gene pool. Genetic and
geologic evidence converge on the theory that there was a catastrophic
die-off of humans about 70,000 years ago caused by a giant volcanic
super eruption in what is now Indonesia.[36] Our species was almost
wiped out by the protracted climate change, and most of us are the
closely related descendants of the few thousand breeding pairs who

survived. Racial differences, for all the trouble they cause, are literally skin deep, of recent vintage, and result in relatively few differences in how medical and mental problems express themselves.

Culture plays a much bigger role but influences only the surface presentations. Brief psychotic disorders and physical symptom presentations are much more common in poorer parts of the world and anorexia nervosa and attention deficit in the richer. In diagnosing and treating, it is crucial to be sensitive to cultural differences, but they are not so great as to require different diagnostic systems for different parts of the world. Across the board, humans are alike enough genetically and culturally that one diagnostic system (either *DSM* or ICD) is elastic enough to fit all the possibilities.

Defining the Individual Mental Disorders

The bad news that we can't develop a useful definition for the general concept "mental disorder" is balanced by the very good news that we can quite easily define each one of the specific mental disorders. The method, introduced by *DSM-III* in 1980, is simple and effective. The description of each *DSM* disorder is accompanied by a criteria set that lists in fairly precise terms which symptoms define it, how many must be present, and their required duration. For example, a major depressive episode is defined as five or more of the following symptoms, presenting together for more than two weeks and causing clinically significant distress or impairment: depressed mood; loss of interest; reduced appetite; changed sleep; fatigue; agitation; guilt; trouble thinking; and suicidal feelings. Clinicians everywhere have been using this as a consensus definition for more than thirty years. Clinical depression is not diagnosed if there are only four instead of five of these very same symptoms, or if they are present for only one week, not two, or if the impairment they cause is not all that big a deal. There are about two hundred criteria sets in the *DSM*—one for each disorder. These establish the boundaries that separate the mental disorders from one another and from normality. Each criteria set has the symptoms that define that particular disorder (panic, generalized anxiety, obsessive-compulsive, attention deficit, autism, etc.) and the required threshold. When clinicians follow the criteria, they achieve reasonable agreement. Without them, there is poor agreement. Each clinician becomes a law unto himself, and the result is a confusing Babel of clashing, idiosyncratic voices.

But there is a catch. The boundaries demarcating the different disorders are ever so much fuzzier in real life than they appear to be on paper. There is really nothing magical or preordained about any of the *DSM* thresholds—shades of gray exist between their seemingly black and white cutoff points. Requiring five symptoms and two weeks for major depressive disorder derives from a fairly arbitrary choice, not a scientific necessity. Just as easily, the set points could have been set higher—say at six symptoms and four weeks. With a more demanding threshold, we would lose in "sensitivity" (thereby missing some sick people who are in need of diagnosis) but would gain in "specificity" (mislabeling fewer normal people). Sensitivity and specificity are reciprocally intertwined—you can't help one without hurting the other. There is an inevitable trade-off between them that requires a proper balancing of the risks and benefits of overdiagnosis versus underdiagnosis. The final decision where to set the bar is always a judgment call; the research never renders a clear and compelling answer forcing the choice of one particular threshold in preference to other possibilities.

Once a criteria set is established, there should be good reasons for changing it; otherwise the system will be not only arbitrary, but also inconsistent and confusing. But this leads to a problem. Many of our current categories and thresholds were created thirty-five years ago when achieving sensitivity was the more important goal—too many people who needed a diagnosis were being missed. Circumstances have now changed dramatically, and poor specificity is now the biggest issue. Before *DSM-III*, there were too few diagnoses—now, because of diagnosis inflation, there are far too many. Raising severity and duration thresholds would help "save normal" and cure excessive diagnosis—but would create instability and reduce sensitivity. You can't have it both ways.

The method of defining disorders by criteria sets has another inherent set of difficult-to-balance trade-offs—between "reliability" and "validity." Reliability means agreement and consistency—will different clinicians seeing the same patient arrive at the same diagnosis. Validity means truth—will the diagnosis tell you what you want to know. Ideally, of course, the definition of a disorder would do both—be both reliable and valid. But to meet the goal of reliability, the defining symptoms must be extremely simple, obvious, and generalize easily across all the people with that particular disorder. If the criteria set includes items that are inferential or complicated, different clinicians will disagree on whether or not they are present. Worshiping at the temple of reliability, the *DSM* criteria sets are as simple as they can be—a catalog only of what is most surface and common in mental disorders. This was a necessary choice, but it necessarily compromises validity—constraining ourselves to the simple blinds us to subtlety, nuance, and individual variability. A great deal is lost in the translation between the rich diversity of different individual experiences of depression and the bland five-of-nine criteria set chosen to define it. In describing the characteristics shared by those who meet the criteria for a given mental disorder, the *DSM* definitions must obscure the ways they are individual and different. *DSM* definitions do not include personal and contextual factors, such as whether the depressive symptoms are an understandable response to a loss, a terrible life situation, psychological conflict, or personality factors.

DSM has to stay simple, but psychiatry doesn't. *DSM* diagnosis should be seen as just one small part of an overall evaluation that would also comprehensively account for the more complicated and individual aspects of each patient. Unfortunately, the *DSM* approach has been far too influential—dominating the field in a way we never intended. Nuanced psychiatry has become checklist psychiatry, homogenizing individual differences and custom-tailored treatments. Psychiatry, once too idiosyncratic and chaotic, has become too standardized and simpleminded. Training programs focus excessive attention on teaching diagnosis and not enough on understanding everything else about the patient.[37] People forget the wisdom of Hippocrates: "It is more important to know what sort of person has a disease than to know what sort of disease a person has." Of course, best practice is to pay close attention to both. *DSM* diagnosis has a necessary place in every evaluation, but it never tells the whole story.

Then there is the problem of knowing which criteria to choose and pretesting for their safety. Before we go prime time with a criteria set, the safe play is to audition it in a field trial. A test drive reduces uncertainty about how it will eventually perform, reducing the risk of unpleasant surprises and the dangers of unwanted fads. The idea is to have clinicians try out the new definition under conditions that approximate real-life circumstances. If the proposal performs well, it becomes official; if poorly, it is revised or scrapped. But again there is a catch. Really several different catches.

First, even the best field trial is performed in the present and can't fully anticipate the future. The carefully done *DSM-IV* attention deficit predicted that our proposed changes would cause only a 15 percent increase in rates. This was probably a fairly accurate estimate given the reality when the data were gathered in the early 1990s. We couldn't foresee the abrupt switch in this reality that occurred in 1997, when drug companies brought new and expensive medicine for ADD to market and were simultaneously set free to advertise them directly to parents and teachers. Soon the selling of ADHD as a diagnosis was ubiquitous in magazines, on your TV screen, and in pediatricians' offices—an unexpected epidemic was born, and the rates of ADHD tripled.

Next, there is the problem of generalizability. The best setting for doing field trials would be the offices of the clinical psychiatrists and of the primary care physicians who actually write most of the prescriptions for psychiatric drugs. But because it is easier, field-testing is instead done in samples of convenience drawn from university research clinics that are very unlike the sites of eventual greatest misuse. The results generated in these cloistered settings will always be much better than what will be obtained in the hustle and bustle of the real world. Then there is the distorting effect of observing the thing observed. It is inherently impossible to learn everything about an electron because the act of observing an electron changes its momentum. Similarly, the act of observing everyday diagnostic practice distorts it so that it is no longer everyday. The selection and training of the clinicians, and their focused attention, make them better diagnosticians within a study than they will be outside of one.

Patient selection in a field trial also artificially raises reliability. In real life, making a diagnosis is like finding a needle in a haystack containing hundreds of possible choices. The field test presents a much easier challenge to the clinician. He knows he is selecting from among only a handful of different choices. Bottom line: Field trials are absolutely necessary but extremely fallible. New suggestions will perform much better in the trial than in real life. Possible future misuses may be entirely undetectable and unpredictable. At their best, field trials will help you avoid some, but certainly not all, the possible future trouble spots.

One final interesting question: Should we use names or numbers in defining mental disorders? The *DSM* system uses only names. Psychologists have developed thousands of rating scales that instead use numbers. Which is better? Like most things, there is no one right answer—it depends on your purpose. Numbers are much more accurate than names—that's why we use them to measure height, weight, IQ, or wavelength in physics. When describing someone's place on a graded continuum, it is ever so much more precise to give a number than a name. "He is six feet tall" saves information lost if the description is reduced simply to "He is tall." Computers love numbers. And so do the researchers who use them.

But most people think names, not numbers. Evolutionary pressures shaped our minds to give simple names, not to make fine-grained mathematical distinctions. We are adapted to a world that required quickly choosing between a yes or no—trying to quantify predators too closely might get you eaten. It's no surprise that statistics as a branch of mathematics arose so late in the game—just a few hundred years ago.

In everyday life, we still usually prefer names to numbers—even though names are admittedly inexact and we do have eager computers ready to crunch whatever numbers we throw at them. We label a color "red" (rather than calling out its exact wavelength) because this is quicker, easier, clearer, and usually serves the purpose. A vivid name, not a confusing bunch of numbers, remains much more convenient for most tasks and provides a clearer and more readily understood image. Clinicians are busy people who have thought in names every step of their natural lives and in all their training. They will not switch to numbers easily, and patients wouldn't understand them if they did. Computer-assisted dimensional diagnosis is certainly the wave of the future, but it is premature and impossible to implement in the present. For now, we will stick to naming the mental disorders, not numbering them.

At the extremes, the distinction between the completely well and the clearly sick is perfectly plain and not the least bit amenable to fudging. In contrast, the much fuzzier distinction between the mildly ill and the probably well is easily and frequently manipulated. Most normal people have at least occasional mild and transitory symptoms (e.g., sadness, anxiety, sleeplessness, sexual dysfunction, substance use) that can easily be misconstrued as mental disorder. The business model of the pharmaceutical industry depends on extending the realm of illness—using creative marketing to expand the pool of customers by convincing the probably well that they are at least mildly sick.

Disease mongering is the fine art of selling psychiatric ills as the most efficient way of peddling very profitable psychiatric pills. Manipulating the market is particularly easy in the United States because we are the only country in the entire world that allows drug companies the freedom to advertise directly to consumers.

Disease mongering cannot occur in a vacuum—it requires that the drug companies engage the active collaboration of the doctors who write the prescriptions, the patients who ask for them, the researchers who invent the new mental disorders, the consumer groups that advocate for more treatment, and the media and Internet that spread the word. A persistent, pervasive, and well-financed "disease awareness" campaign can create disease where none existed before. And psychiatry is especially vulnerable to manipulation of the normal/disease boundary because it lacks biological tests and relies heavily on subjective judgments that can be easily influenced by clever marketing.

The primary loyalty of any corporation is to its shareholders and to its own-survival, not to the public weal. General Motors sells cars, Anheuser-Busch sells beer, Apple sells computers, the drug cartels sell cocaine, and drug companies sell pills all for the same reason—to generate as big a profit as possible. The profitability of any corporation depends on increasing the size of its market and its margins on each sale. Drug companies are exemplary profit-making machines because of their highly developed skill in pushing product and their ability to maintain monopoly pricing. Pumping up diagnostic inflation is absolutely key to drug company success. Full saturation requires having the widest demographic reach, from the youngest child to the oldest adult. Casting the broadest net is always great for shareholders, but is very often bad news for the mislabeled normals who are subjected to the unnecessary medication and stigma that comes with fake diagnosis.

Is Normality Resilient or Fragile?

The paradoxical answer is both. Resiliency is built into every aspect of our biological, psychological, and social being. We are hardwired to work remarkably well, but are far too complicated always to work perfectly and we can lose purchase on normality by mislabeling as mental disorder each and every one of our glitches.

The governing principle of all of life is "homeostasis"—a portmanteau word that combines the Greek terms "homeo" (same) with "stasis" (stable) to doubly emphasize the pursuit of equilibrium. At every level from the single cell to the entire society, nature constantly seeks to compensate for all perturbations and to reestablish stable balance to return to whatever is the normal or expectable range of function. Systems don't survive very long unless they can achieve homeostasis in the face of both external and internal challenges and disruptions. Each of our cells is a complex and hardworking factory whose survival depends on maintaining the proper metabolic balance of millions of chemical interactions. Each organ is a collaboration of cells and our body is a collaboration of organs, each dependent for its survival on the balanced functioning of all the others. Homeostasis is what keeps our body temperature, blood pressure, and pulse rate stable. Our body is a constant wonder of billions of trade-offs.

In the interpersonal realm, marriages end in divorce if they lack the homeostatic gift of smoothing the rough edges of inevitable conflict. In the political realm, states that can't find homeostatic balance among competing forces suffer civil war or collapse. Homeostasis also governs any inanimate physical or chemical processes that are in a prolonged steady state. We would not have our comfortable home in this solar system were it not in a state of gentle homeostatic equilibrium—a delicate balance that we are now threatening by pollution and overpopulation.

Any failure of homeostasis in an animate system leads to malfunction, disease, and eventually (if severe and prolonged enough) death.

Cancer, diabetes, hypertension, heart failure, obesity, and most other illnesses all represent the breakdown of homeostatic feedback mechanisms that normally keep our bodies in balance. And medical treatments for illness all have in common the aim of restoring an internal balance that has been lost in the face of disease.

The human brain is our world's grandest expression of homeostasis. It is the master regulator of most of our bodily functions and also a master at regulating that most complex of all machines—itself. Our thoughts, emotions, and behaviors are the final result of an indescribably complex coordination of billions of cells firing off in a carefully tuned, exquisite equilibrium. No computer engineer would have the audacity (much less the ability) to create something so complex—too many things could go wrong along the way. And doubtless they do. But nature has found the means to provide good enough wiring and compensatory balance most of the time. Brain homeostasis has sufficient resources and redundancies to react to internal and external challenges, bringing things back to normal and keeping us functioning pretty much within the straight and narrow.

We are hardy survivors—men and women for all seasons, built to work in all climates, to eat every conceivable food and to survive long periods without food, to fight battles and to run away, to love and to hate, to feel a wide gamut of emotions, and to evince a startling array of different behaviors. We are not only much alike but also preserve specialized individual differences essential for the survival of the small groups that endured the rigors of the past hundreds of thousands of years. The tribe needed the proper balance of many individual capacities—it would not do well with all leaders or all followers, with all warriors or all pacifists, if everyone was paranoid or gullible.

We can feel sadness, grief, worry, anger, disgust, and terror because these are all adaptive. At times (especially in response to interpersonal, psychological, and practical stresses), our emotions may temporarily get out of hand and cause considerable distress or impairment. But homeostasis and time are great natural healers, and most people resiliently right themselves and regain their normal balance. Psychiatric disorder consists of symptoms and behaviors that are not self-correcting—a breakdown in the normal homeostatic healing process. Diagnostic inflation occurs when we confuse the typical perturbations that are part of everyone's life with true psychiatric disorder (which is relatively uncommon, perhaps affecting 5 to 10 percent of the population at any given time).

Mental disorders should be diagnosed only when the presentation is clear-cut, severe, and clearly not going away on its own. The best way to deal with the everyday problems of living is to solve them directly or to wait them out, not to medicalize them with a psychiatric diagnosis or treat them with a pill. Prematurely resorting to medication short-circuits the traditional pathways of restorative natural healing—seeking support from family, friends, and the community; making needed life changes, off-loading excessive stress; pursuing hobbies and interests, exercise, rest, distraction, a change of pace. Overcoming problems on your own normalizes the situation, teaches new skills, and brings you closer to the people who were helpful. Taking a pill labels you as different and sick, even if you really aren't. Medication is essential when needed to reestablish homeostasis for those who are suffering from real psychiatric disorder. Medication interferes with homeostasis for those who are suffering from the problems of everyday life.

A study we did twenty-five years ago taught me an unforgettable lesson about human resilience. It was at the height of the AIDS epidemic and before there were any effective treatments. Getting a positive test result was then the equivalent of a death sentence—and a very unpleasant death at that. We found that men who tested positive had an immediate large jump in measures of sadness and anxiety—no surprise, given the fatal implications of the test. Men who tested negative had a smaller, but still large, reduction in these same measures—again no surprise that they would be greatly relieved. Really amazing were the scores six weeks later. Both groups had returned pretty much to their baselines—the HIV positives were resiliently dealing with their really terrible news; the HIV negatives did not get a permanent mood lift from their really wonderful news. Homeostasis had brought both groups back to where they started. Had we immediately jumped in with medication to treat the painful symptoms in the positives, we would have interfered with their natural healing and given them another burden to add to the ones they already had. The lesson is clear—we have far too much faith in pills, far too little trust in resilience, time, and homeostasis.

Normal Is Fuzzy and Therefore Fragile

"Normal" and mental disorder turn out to be a frustratingly elusive—inherently incapable of anything resembling clear, bright-line definition. The realm of the "normal" has been rapidly shrinking as an expanding psychiatry stretches easily across its elastic boundary. Are my son's temper tantrums part of growing up or an early sign of bipolar disorder? Does my daughter's inattentiveness at school mean she has attention deficit disorder or is she just extra smart and bored with the dull stuff being covered there? Should I be pleased by my son's precocious interest in rockets and science fiction or worried that he is autistic? Am I experiencing expectable worries and sadness or is this generalized anxiety disorder? If I don't remember a face or a fact, is Alzheimer's just around the corner? Is grief a useful, inevitable, and poignant sign of my broken heart, or is it a major depressive disorder? Is my teenage daughter a creative eccentric, or a psychotic-to-be who needs a dangerous drug? Is Tiger Woods a mental patient or a philanderer? Is a brutal rapist simply bad or possibly mad? All of us have mild and transient psychiatric symptoms from time to time—does this mean we are all flirting with mental illness?

Questions about what's normal and what causes abnormal have been with us since the dawn of man. Our ancestors found creative answers that always made good sense to them at the time. Some now seem brilliantly intuitive, others daffy, and a few were positively diabolical. A quick detour through this past will help us understand the present and avoid mistakes in the future.

CHAPTER 2

From Shaman to Shrink

History doesn't repeat itself, but it sure does rhyme.
MARK TWAIN

Man is the naming animal—we can't stop ourselves from putting a label on everything in sight. This has been our special gift, and sometimes our curse, ever since Genesis, when Adam established his dominion over the plants and animals by the simple act of naming them.[1] Diagnostic exuberance is built into our DNA. We have a strong need to identify patterns—to distinguish lion from lamb, food from poison, friend from foe.

Almost as important was psychiatric diagnosis. Abnormal behavior has always threatened our survival because we are so dependent on tribal harmony. We need a name and an explanation as a way of gaining control over actions that threaten the individual and the social group (whether these occur on the savanna or at the office). Labeling was and remains an important way of reducing uncertainty and providing a sense of (often false) mastery. Finding patterns helps sort untidy experience into manageable units—an inexact or incorrect name or explanation for mental disorder beats having none at all.

And man is not satisfied with mere naming. The natural next steps are grouping the names into categories; then the categories into a classification; and finally trying to figure out an explanation for why things sort as they do. Of course, the specific explanations have varied greatly over time. Formerly, they were the stuff of religion and folklore; now the same curiosity and need for order drives our search for scientific understanding. What seem now to be fanciful myths were once the best science of the time, and our current best science will itself in the not-too-distant future be seen as no more than fanciful myth.

The labeling of mental disorder has evolved over time because the lens of cultural attention extracts figure from ground in many different ways. We see elephants in clouds if we look for them, but could equally well find whales or rabbits if these better fit our preconceptions—the cloud doesn't have to change for people to see different shapes in it. Psychiatric diagnosis is seeing something that exists, but with a pattern shaped by what we expect to see. Because there is no one right way, fashions prevail. The ancient shaman had different names and explanations—but these worked almost as well for him as current names and explanations work for the modern shrink. Understanding our current methods of psychiatric diagnosis requires that we make a quick study of how we got here.

The Shaman and the Spirit World

Psychiatry seems like a young profession, barely two hundred years old, but you could fairly say it is the oldest. Diagnosing and ministering to the mentally ill was part of the job description of the shaman, or medicine man. He (often she) was a tribe's first paid professional, the only person to have a specialized role outside the round of hunting and gathering. While everyone else was off finding food, the shaman got to stay home doing sick call, using his magic to assess the causes and apply the cures for mental and physical symptoms.

Of course, to earn his keep, he had to do lots of other jobs as well. The word *shaman* means "one who knows," and he had to know a lot. He kept the world in balance and the game plentiful. He could reveal the past and predict the future. He memorized the stories telling how the earth began and the tribe was born. He owned the sacred objects and could find magical plant medicines. He led the rituals. The shaman was medicine man, spiritual medium, judge, intellectual, and entertainer. He literally had to sing the tribe's songs for his supper. And he could dance.[2]

But doing psychiatry was always a big part of a shaman's practice. We are social animals whose survival is completely dependent on good relationships and group cohesion. Abnormal behavior constitutes a threat not only to the individual; it is also a clear and present danger to the future of the tribe. Psychiatric emergencies must be quickly labeled, understood, treated, and cured. The shaman had all the tools to define and deal with abnormality. He could diagnose mental disorder, explain its origin, and make it better.

The most popular diagnoses invoked a malevolent spirit, a mischievous curse, or a broken taboo. The treatment required entering the spirit world with trance, vision quest, or dream work, perhaps facilitated by a psychedelic mushroom or plant. Healing rituals included singing, dancing, fasting, sweating, and sleep deprivation. The shaman would invite the patient to leave the everyday world and temporarily enter his magic circle. They would fight with or cajole the spirits until a deal was brokered so that all could be well again. The shaman had great authority and healing power.[3] Magical belief and suggestion can go a long way. But beyond the hocus-pocus, he had practical common sense, wisdom about human nature, and medicinal plants. Cures were expensive, and the shaman was the richest person in the tribe.

The Priests and the Gods

The domestication of plants and animals in the last ten thousand years gave man greater control over the natural world and a larger sense of his place in it. Nature animism never completely disappeared but was partially replaced by the birth of a pantheon of gods who (though gifted with immortality and extraordinary powers) seemed otherwise to speak and act just like you and me. Amongst agriculturalists, the shaman was as obsolete as a blacksmith is now, replaced by a new professional—the priest (or the priestess). The job descriptions were very different in some ways, similar in others. The shaman had been intermediary to the spirit world. The priest became the intermediary between man and gods, retaining the shaman's magical spirit powers but augmenting them with divine authority. The shaman was mobile and treated people wherever the tribe happened to be that day on its round of nomadic migration—the spirits lived everywhere. Though relatively rich, he could carry his lifelong possessions on his back. In contrast, the priest was sedentary, working out of a temple complex on holy ground consecrated by the gods, usually near a spring of purifying holy water. Befitting the surplus wealth of a prosperous agricultural society, many of these were elegantly appointed facilities with spas, a library, a gymnasium, and a theater.

But, in fundamental ways, the priest's job description was the same as the shaman's. Keep the gods happy and the world in balance; ward off catastrophic punishments; bring on the food. And minister to the ill, among whom were many with problems we would label mental disorder. The priest spent a lot of his time being a shrink.

Greek myth is full of madness, clear evidence that mental disorder has always puzzled us. Whatever man did that seemed beyond himself (either exceeding or failing expectations) was attributed to the action of a divinity. When a hero acted crazy, and many did, the standard diagnosis was "the goddess made him do it." Early on, abnormal behavior was blamed on the goddess named, fittingly enough, Mania—a primal, primitive demon figure who existed before there were men and whose function was to drive them out of their minds. Later the familiar Olympian gods and (more often) goddesses got into the act—with jealous Hera being the most likely crazy-maker.

Why were goddesses so likely to drive men crazy? Woman's rights had taken a big hit when farming and shepherding replaced hunting and gathering. The new power and land-owning relationships greatly favored the patriarchs and their male divinities, making women household furniture. The vengeful goddesses represented the feared forces that had been suppressed in the masculine takeover. Divine wrath was a great excuse for (usually male) bad behavior. Madness was a punishment, but also a way to off-load responsibility—the diagnosis both explained deviant behavior and excused it. If Hercules is murderously destructive, it must be Hera punishing his hubris and impiety. If Ajax is mindlessly slaughtering his cattle, it must be Athena misdirecting his envious anger.

Special gifts were also linked to madness; divine inspiration comes at a price. Cassandra and the priestess at Delphi can see the future, but they must be mad in the present. The Muses often bring madness with their poetry. The cult of Dionysus threw substance abuse into the mix. Wine, sex, and religious frenzy were a way to bring voluntary states of madness that took a person temporarily away from everyday normality and brought him closer to the gods. Normals might also malinger madness: Ulysses unsuccessfully feigned madness to avoid military service at Troy, King David to save his life.

The gods were jealous and whimsical and definitely played favorites. The rules were unclear and unfair. You needed a priest to teach you how to keep the gods on your side and out of your head. He exercised the authority conferred by sacred beliefs, holy prayers, magical rituals, and a grand temple. In the eighth century BCE (at the very time Homer was compiling his songs of Troy), the first medical temple was dedicated to the cult worship of Asclepius, god of healing. You could recognize Asclepius by his distinctive rod with coiled snake, which remains the symbol of medicine. Their ability to shed skin had made snakes terrific models of immortality and healing; harmless ones in large numbers were given the run of the temple grounds. The healing cult thrived. Soon three hundred temples dedicated to Asclepius were consecrated all over ancient Greece, usually sited in remote and beautiful places with a sacred spring or mountain view, or both. For a thousand years the institution was wildly popular and remarkably effective. The Romans adopted it and brought healing temples to the reaches of the empire. The Asclepieia were all-purpose—temple, hospital, hotel, health spa, resort, entertainment center, and medical school —some combination of Lourdes, the Mayo Clinic, and a Ritz-Carlton. Access to the temples required an extended and difficult pilgrimage, impossible for those with severe medical or psychiatric illness. The temples were probably treating a population of patients who presented with a combination of milder physical and emotional symptoms, not very different from many patients seen today in a primary care doctor's office. The pilgrims had proven, by the long hike, that they had high motivation to get better and a profound belief in the cure.

The priests had developed a new theory of mental illness, a new system of diagnosis, and a new treatment. The theory was visitation by angry or jealous gods. The diagnostic procedure, called "incubation," required a meeting of the minds with the god. After being purified, the pilgrim would be permitted the privilege of sleeping near the god's sacred altar in the holiest room of the temple. He was expected to have revelatory dreams or visions that would signify a successful divine visitation. The god might make his message clear and provide an obvious dream or might remain obscure in a confusing one. The temples delivered a treatment that anticipated aspects of psychoanalysis. The priest, dressed in the robes and carrying the rod of Asclepius, was on duty to assist with expert dream interpretation. He would help you discover the meaning of your dream—deciphering the god's message about the nature of your illness, its cause, and the steps needed to placate divine forces. If you couldn't muster a dream or vision of your own, or were too sick or busy to make the trip, there were professional dreamers who did incubation-by-proxy on your behalf.

The full temple experience also included other magical and practical amenities. There were rituals, prayers, incantations, and sacrifices intended to please the gods. The priest also specialized in psychotherapy, commonsensical advice, and medicinal plants. Surgeries were also performed as needed. On top of this there were gym and spa services, diet advice, opportunities for intellectual stimulation at the library, and entertainment at the theater. And there was wine. The high cure rates are not surprising. The patient would be expected to contribute a generous thank-offering to the god. A tablet documenting the miracle cure would be prepared and displayed prominently, among many others. Advertising was good for temple business and heightened the prestige of its healing powers.[4] The healing temple survives today in three very different forms—sacred sites of modern pilgrimage for faith healing; secular spas that promote natural health by exposure to exercise, diet, and beauty; and the modern medical center.

Hippocrates: Father of Medicine (Circa 460 BCE to 370 BCE)

A religious understanding of the world has always been (and probably always will be) man's greatest comfort in adapting to its uncertainties and hardships. Supernatural belief of one sort or another has dominated most times and most places. But the Greeks, beginning in the seventh century BCE, developed an alternative, secular model to explain how the world works and why people get sick. They called it natural philosophy; we call it science. This new method has great explanatory power and creates its own brand of awe and beauty. The worship of unseen supernatural forces was replaced by close observation of the natural world and careful reasoning about the underlying principles that govern its operation.

The Greeks were not working in a vacuum. They synthesized the considerable science base of the Babylonian, Persian, Egyptian, and Indian cultures and extended it on a grand intellectual tour that gave birth to the modern world. The progress was swift and enriched all of human learning. Pythagoras demonstrated that the language of mathematics could systematically describe the secrets of nature. Democritus intuited that the apparent complexity of the universe is reducible to simpler, irreducible atoms. The Greeks knew that Earth is round and revolves around the sun, and accurately calculated its circumference. They even speculated about "multiverses." Euclid devised geometry, and Archimedes devised the beginnings of calculus.

And the Greeks invented modern medicine. Hippocrates introduced a fully biological understanding of mental and medical illness that required no gods, no priestly authority, no sacrifice, and no ritual incantation. "From nothing else but the brain come joys, delights, laughter and sports, and sorrows, griefs, despondency, and lamentations . . . and by the same organ, we become mad and delirious, and fears and terrors assail us . . . all these things we endure from the brain, when it is not healthy." Psychiatric and medical problems came from an imbalance of the four basic "humors": blood, yellow bile, black bile, and phlegm. Cures would come from natural (not supernatural) processes. The physician would necessarily be limited by the biological realities; he could assist but never guarantee cure. He would be better at predicting the prognosis than changing it. But he could always comfort, console, and advise—and these too are crucial to healing.

Medicine (and psychiatry) would take man as its measure and humane treatment as its goal. Healing became a secular profession based exclusively on scientific observation and practical knowledge. Studying his patients closely and taking careful notes, Hippocrates clustered symptoms into many new diseases, each with well-documented course, predictable prognosis, and particular epidemiology. He described mania, melancholia, phrenitis, and phobia. No mysticism of any sort intruded upon diagnosis and treatment. Illness was not a punishment or a visitation of the gods; it was part of nature. "Men regard the nature and cause of disease as divine from ignorance and wonder."

Hippocrates was a genius at prognosis and saw it as the most essential skill in medical practice. He recognized the importance of sorting patients into three groups: those who get better on their own; those who need medical treatment; and those who will not respond to any intervention. This "rule of thirds," the most robust finding in medical history, is still taught to medical students and holds today for many psychiatric disorders.

The treatment recommendation depends on the patient's prognosis. For group one, don't give treatments that may do harm, because they will get better with time and support; for group three, don't give harmful treatments because they will add to the burden of illness without providing cure; instead, provide solace and comfort. Specific treatment should be pursued only for group two, balancing the risks of treatment with those posed by illness. Be sure that interventions are more likely to help than harm. Hippocrates favored cautious, mild, natural healing except when extreme circumstances required and justified a more aggressive approach. He would be puzzled and deeply saddened by the promiscuous use of harmful antipsychotic medicine that has become a dangerous part of current practice.

Hippocrates was a modest man, loving toward and beloved by his patients and students. Never doctrinaire or authoritarian, he took pleasure in learning from accumulated clinical experience, his own and others. He institutionalized the concept of secular medical education and practice—of learning at the bedside. His students further developed his methods and created a distinctive style of clear and objective medical writing.[5] An interesting sidebar is that Thucydides borrowed from the Hippocratic style in his great clinical descriptions of the sickness that is our human history.

Galen: Father of Personality Theory (AD 130 to AD 200)

Galen was a man for all medical seasons—a healer of bodies and mender of minds. No doctor ever had a wider clinical experience, investigated such varied diseases, invented more treatments, or wrote so many words.[6] When he wasn't busy being team doctor for a stable of gladiators, inventing cataract surgery, and performing brain operations not repeated till modern times, Galen expanded the scope of humoral theory to explain human personality and its impact on illness. The humors explained not just what ails us but also who we are. Our fate is not determined by our stars or by the demons or the gods—instead it is based on the balance of our bodily chemistries. This biological model of temperament and its effect on behavior is not very different from modern theories, except that he got the specific chemistries wrong.

The Greeks did things in fours. There were four seasons, four ages of life, four planets, and there were four elements (air, fire, earth, and water) that in various combinations determined the physics of the world and the biology of body and mind. There were four humors (blood, yellow bile, black bile, and phlegm), each related to one of the elements. Hippocrates had noted that an imbalance of these causes illness. Galen added to the standard system that personality also comes from an imbalance of these same humors. Too much blood produced an excessively sanguine personality; too much yellow bile, the choleric; too much black bile, the melancholic; too much phlegm, the phlegmatic. Their harmonious balance led to normal mental functioning. There were all possible permutations of various mixes of humors that explained and gave color to the great variety of human behavior and tendencies. All this sounds "quackish" now, but it governed medicine for more than fifteen hundred years. For comparison, the half-life of many current theories is measured in decades, not centuries.

By temperament, Galen meant not only the behavioral aspects of personality but also its bodily manifestations. Mind and body were interacting; personality and health were inextricably linked. You could predict how a person of a given temperamental mix would behave, but you could also predict how his body would behave—which illnesses he was most likely to get and which treatments would work. Illnesses might come and go but your temperament was inborn and fairly stable. It could be influenced and brought into balance with appropriate interventions—diet, activity, herbs, bloodletting, cupping, purging. The treatment had to be very individualized, since there were so many permutations of imbalance among the four humors.

Galen understood that brain dysfunction and mental illness could have many causes (environmental or constitutional) other than an imbalance of the humors. Wine could drive man mad. His experience with the gladiators taught him the importance of head trauma, and the causative role of brain fevers was obvious. He also recognized that mental retardation was due to congenital problems in brain functioning. Equivalent to current practice, before making a diagnosis of personality disorder, one had to rule out the possibility that medical illnesses or substance use was responsible for the person's behavior. Only when there was no more definite cause would temperament and humoral balance be considered primary.

Treating humoral imbalance was a balancing act that first required a careful diagnosis to determine which fluid was tipping the scales and then changing the patient's life to even things out. Vomits, purges, sweats, and bleeding were obvious because of their direct impact on the fluids. Various herbs, spices, metals, hot and cold, dry and wet, were believed to have differential medicinal impacts that could titrate each humor. Curative manipulations included baths, climate change, and diet. There was also a philosophy-of-living component—each person has a very individualized temperament that will do best and be healthiest within a particular way of life. Once the temperament is diagnosed, a next step is to determine which aspects of the person's life upset balance, which provide support. The prescription would be an adjustment in environment and daily habits (study, work, diet, sex, drinking, music, family relations) to correct the fluid imbalance and thereby improve personality, increase happiness, and prevent medical illness.

Galen dominated medicine for much longer than he should have or would have wanted to. Later generations accepted his writings as doctrine, honoring his authority but failing to honor his methods of independent observation and experiment. The humoral theory wasn't conclusively overturned until the mid-1800s, when Virchow demonstrated the role played by the cell in disease. But Galen's insight that inborn tendencies in personality affect mental and physical illness is as fresh as the day it was born.

The Dark Age of Demons

The treatment of the mentally ill in Europe went into the Dark Ages, which lasted from the fall of Rome (in the fifth century) to the rise of Philippe Pinel (in the late eighteenth). The dark ages were never nearly so benighted as we imagine (and there were always isolated bright spots), but for the mentally ill this was the worst of times, the worst of places. The Greek biological theories recognized the humanity of the mentally ill and regarded their strange behaviors as fully understandable within a medical model. The mentally ill were people like us who happened to have a biological imbalance. Not their fault and not scary, just unfortunate.

The Greek medical enlightenment was a victim of the Dark Ages. The doctor of medicine who diagnosed chemical imbalance was replaced by the doctor of the church who diagnosed demonic possession. Exorcism, inquisition, torture, and the stake replaced medical treatment. The mentally ill were inhabited by dangerously contagious, demonic forces that had to be destroyed as part of God's struggle against the devil. Certainly there were exceptions (kindnesses extended and hospitals built by religious orders), but overall the treatment of the mentally ill was a holocaust and a shameful chapter in the history of the Church. Christian theology, mixed with pagan demonology, created a story line depicting mental illness as the devil's handiwork. The moral neutrality of humoral theory was no match for a vivid religious drama portraying an eternal battle of God versus Devil, with madmen (and more often madwomen) as pawns on the losing side.

The Western world equated difference with evil and feared its contagion. Someone acting strange could be communing with the devil and threatening the welfare (and eternal salvation) of the entire community. In extreme cases, torture and execution were considered fully justifiable as part of God's work. In milder cases, recovery was possible, but only after a confession of sin and a willingness to return to God and holiness. Greek scientific observation was replaced by a quaint system of spiritual diagnosis that matched the peculiarity of different mental states with a hierarchy of different devils. A pall of religious delusion had settled on Europe that sanctified a mean-spirited cruelty in the treatment of its most vulnerable citizens.[7]

Death did not protect the mentally ill from continued indignity. In canon law, attempting suicide was a crime instigated by the devil to spite God. The corpse was a fit candidate for extended punishment that might consist of some combination of hanging, torture, mutilation, and being dragged through the streets. Survivors of suicide attempts might expect to have their death wish fulfilled by superstitious neighbors, often in the cruelest way, to ensure that their devils were properly punished. The prohibition against burial in consecrated ground extended the punishment into eternity.

The *Malleus Maleficarum*, published in 1487, codified demonic doctrine and provided rationale and legal force for an inquisition of the mentally ill.[8] They were weeded out with brutally efficient and inhumanly cruel bureaucratic methods. The mad were judged by God and man to be witches and demons, deserving no mercy and (with few exceptions) receiving none.

In more enlightened religious circles, sin gradually replaced possession as the diagnosis of choice and explanation of mental disorder.

Disagreeable behaviors and manners were the outward symptoms of an unruly, uncivilized, greedy, and lascivious nature. The mentally ill had graduated from being demons to being sinners. Their behavior reflected not the direct intervention of the devil, but rather the immoral and ungoverned exercise of their own free will. In this they were not very different from the common criminals with whom they were often enough housed. Harsh treatment was recommended to redirect the mentally ill to the straight and narrow of passions governed and sins renounced. They needed to be taken in hand, tamed, and restrained. Sinful natures were stubborn and ingrained. Some of the treatment consisted of moral suasion; much of it was physical punishment. There were attempts to enhance the spiritual life of the mentally ill and to teach them habits of order, self-discipline, and restraint. This was intended to bring them closer to God and away from sin. But for the recalcitrant sinner who refused to get better under the direction of this light-handed approach, punishment had to be commensurately severe. Spare the rod and spoil the patient. The illness had to be quelled along with the sinful pride that caused it; morality was instilled with a strong hand that included all manner of physical restraint, whipping and other corporal punishments, spinning chairs, freezing baths, and other forms of exposure. Though punitive in the extreme by modern standards, such treatment was not as unrestrained in its cruelty or lethal in its effect as when it had been directed at the devil or his agent. No longer used were the torture tools of the inquisitorial trade or burning at the stake. The mad were seen as bad and treated as such, but at least they were not personifications of the devil.

Certainly there were important exceptions to Europe's dark treatment of the mad. Many Christian charity hospitals were founded in the thirteenth century in monasteries and on the stops to the holy land or pilgrimage sites. The mad, the physically ill, lepers, orphans, and the poor were given room, board, prayers, and Christian understanding by monks and nuns. Therapy was minimal, scientific observation and clinical diagnosis nil. The goal was Christian care, not diagnosis or cure. But this was a huge step up from the stake.

But the more naturalistic, biological view was never completely suppressed. Humoral medicine had always kept a slender foothold in the monasteries and was greatly revived during the Crusades when rude Western invaders encountered the much more advanced medical civilization of the Muslim world. Galen's treatises that had previously been translated from Greek to Arabic were now translated from Arabic to Latin. Town universities began to replace monasteries as centers of learning, and each established a medical faculty with a naturalistic worldview that to some degree balanced the demonology of its theology department. The professors of medicine taught that natural, humoral causes of madness should be considered exclusions before assuming demonic possession. Unfortunately, the impact of the professors on practice was negligible. Medicine was taught as theory only, and its teachers were ivory tower types who spoke with Galen's authority, but had no patients. Without close personal observation, it was impossible for them to have much influence or to advance the clinical science of understanding mental illness. Indeed, the naturalistic purpose of the medical professors was sometimes perverted to the cause of theorizing on the physiology of demonic possession and how it affected sanity. One interesting side effect of Galen's renewed influence was a dramatic increase in the price of the treasured spices that had to be imported from the Orient; these were seen as particularly useful medicines in regulating the body humors.

Even in an age of superstition, common sense and humane attitudes never totally disappeared. Not every problem was demonized, not every patient subjected to torture. Other factors—overwork, overeating, too much sex, or excessive worry—were sometimes considered causative and called for reasonable treatment, behavioral changes, prayer, pilgrimages, rituals, and amulets. Many were cured through "miracles of faith." And exorcisms did not all require trauma or death;

sometimes they were symbolic—a model of the devil, not the person, would be beaten.

The Arabs Invent Modern Psychiatry (Circa AD 700 to AD 1500)

Before entering its own dark age five centuries ago, the Arab world was the undisputed center of knowledge and progress. Islam had initially welcomed the wonders of scientific discovery as a way of perceiving Allah and his intentions. Current tribal readings of the Koran run directly counter to the intellectual freedom it had offered from the time of Mohammed until the clerics gained control as Arab political power waned in the sixteenth century. The Arabs were the first people in the world to introduce quantitative experimental science, taking advantage of their convenient number system (now ours), which greatly facilitated the computations that were so tedious using Roman numerals. They invented algebra, spherical geometry, and trigonometry. They preserved and integrated the best of Greek, Indian, and Persian science and expanded them all with native genius.

Along the way, the Arabs invented psychiatry as a discipline and psychiatrists as a separate specialty and brought psychiatry to a level of sophistication in diagnosis, treatment, and theory not seen in Europe until the nineteenth century. Why the Arabs? The Koran has an enlightened view of mental illness, with none of the denigrating demonology of the Judeo-Christian and Greco-Roman traditions. No angry spirits, no jealous gods. Mental illness was a practical problem to be dealt with on human and humane terms, with no supernatural blinders.

The Koran enjoins "feed and clothe the insane . . . and tell splendid words to him." It sensibly advised against allowing the severely mentally ill to make property decisions, but it insisted that they be treated well and with respect. This led to a totally secular, enlightened, and clinical approach. The mentally ill were to receive custodial care in well-run hospitals whose mission was also to document and understand their problems. The first hospital specifically for the mentally ill opened in Baghdad in 705; Cairo followed in 800; and soon many other major cities. Muslim hospitals often employed Jewish and Christian doctors and included large outpatient clinics and pharmacies.

The progression of psychiatric advance was astounding and anticipates exactly the same steps that occurred a millennium later when separate asylums for the mentally ill were finally established in Europe. The mental hospital was a wonderful cradle for scientific discovery. The psychiatric specialists had intimate access to a wide variety of patients and could compare their different courses over the passage of time. They made accurate clinical observations, sorted symptoms into syndromes, and developed effective treatment approaches. Arab psychiatry attained a level of detailed, practical learning never before known in the world and not to be achieved again until about 1900.

A variety of psychiatric classifications were devised in the same excited way as occurred under similar circumstances in the West during the nineteenth century. The Arab world created a completely workable description of disorders equivalent to a modern *DSM*. Severity was divided into levels that were equivalent to later concepts of neurosis and psychosis. Depression was divided into endogenous, reactive, agitated, and involutional. There were good descriptions of mania, delirium, dementia, epilepsy, meningitis, and stroke. Delusions, hallucinations, strange behavior, and poor judgment were grouped into something like schizophrenia. Phobias, obsessions, compulsions, impotence, sleep disorder, hypochondriasis, and lovesickness were recognized. Clearly the basic psychiatric disorders are stable over time—even if fads come and go.

Careful brain dissection disproved some of Galen's assertions and revealed the distributions of the cerebral nerves and vasculature. Tracing the sensory tracts localized the different brain locations for sensory perception. It was known that the frontal lobe was needed for reasoning and common sense and that the ventricles expand in dementia.

Arab psychiatry anticipated the holistic and respectful moral treatment that didn't reach Europe for another thousand years. While patients were being scourged, tortured, and burned in the West, they received wise counseling, cognitive psychotherapy, dream interpretation, drugs, baths, music, and work therapy in the East. Mental and physical health were seen as closely intertwined; each could affect the other. The Arabs also accumulated a body of sophisticated knowledge on cognitive psychology, perception, psychotherapy, and neuroscience.[9]

Sydenham Spots Syndromes

Living at the dawn of the Enlightenment in seventeenth-century Cromwellian England, Thomas Sydenham retaught Europe the Hippocratic natural history method of medicine and psychiatry—no demons and no dogmas and no devilishly dangerous treatments. It is from patients that we learn disease, not theory or philosophy or religious doctrine. With his friend the philosopher John Locke, he developed an empirical, atheoretical approach to knowledge acquisition. Sydenham was the prince of practical, commonsense medicine. "You must go to the bedside. It is there alone you can learn disease." The art of medicine could properly be learned only from its practice and its patients.

Sydenham's special role was to bring nosology, which is the classification of diseases, back to the center of medical attention. He was a master at describing syndromes and diseases. Observe, analyze, and compare. Identify regularly cooccurring clusters of symptoms and study their course and prognosis. Diseases were like plants or animals in the way they could be distinguished from one another—if only you know how to look and looked long and hard enough. Ultimately, understanding the pattern will help you uncover the cause and discover the treatment. "Nature, in the production of disease, is uniform and consistent, so much so, that for the same disease in different persons the symptoms are for the most part the same; and the selfsame phenomena that you would observe in the sickness of Socrates you would observe in the sickness of a simpleton."

Among the many diseases Sydenham studied and nailed were hysteria and hypochondriasis. Unlike the more gullible Charcot and Freud, working two hundred years later, Sydenham recognized that patients presenting with the physical symptoms of psychological distress could often be made worse by overtreatment. Stopping extreme treatments and substituting psychological techniques often helped patients recover. "Sometimes I have consulted my patients' safety and my own reputation most effectually by doing nothing at all."

Seventeenth-century England, awash in plagues, was a wonderful laboratory for studying the spread of fevers. Sydenham was a pioneer in epidemiology, again following the model of Hippocrates, who had invented the field. Understanding the environmental causes of disease and contagions is the basis of a preventive public health approach that is much more effective than treating their consequences.

Sydenham took the mystery out of chorea—contractions of the limbs and trunk that are outside the person's control. He pointed out that chorea occurred after a strep throat, as did rheumatic fever—brain inflammation caused the movements, not demons. He also made three revolutionary and enduring contributions to the drug treatment of diseases: using the extract of a Peruvian bark that happened to contain quinine to treat malaria; promoting iron for anemia; and preparing a liquid form of opium, a medicine he much admired. But Sydenham was cautious in his prescription habits and suspicious of the heroically harmful treatment zealotry of many of his colleagues.[10]

Linnaeus Shows That Classification Counts

It would have been fun to have lived in the eighteenth century. This self-described period of "Enlightenment" was the one moment in history when it was most reasonable to hope that the steady advance of human knowledge would lead to our happiness. But the century ended badly and crushed illusions that have been impossible to resuscitate since. The French Revolution and Napoleonic wars burst the bubble of innocence. Subsequent experience revealed what previously unimaginable disasters can follow from human knowledge when it is unguided by wisdom and caution.

But a smart person living in the 1700s (there were many) could still believe in the eventual perfectibility of man and the world. It was just a question of gathering data and finding the right way of ordering it. Astronomy provided a seductively simple model of science solving nature's riddles. First came the Copernican descriptive theory of a solar-centered universe. Then painstaking observations by Brahe and mathematical sorting of data points by Kepler. And finally, the great triumph of human understanding. Newton (with a big assist from Galileo) explains not only the grand motions of the stars and planets, but also what keeps our feet stuck on the ground and why a cannonball hits a target. Newton's synthesis challenged science to seek basic truths in other intellectual pursuits. There was a feverish search for new knowledge and for better ways of sorting it. The enlightenment became the Age of Taxonomy, and the daddy of all classifiers was Carl Linnaeus.

Among the many appealing geniuses of the Enlightenment, Linnaeus is my personal favorite. He was a practicing physician and a fervent botanist, then a necessary combination of roles. Since the days of the shaman, most useful medicines have come from plants, and every medical school was centered on its garden. Linnaeus never personally collected specimens beyond northern Europe, but he didn't have to. The world came to him. His students were encouraged to become "apostles" pursuing adventure and specimens as ships' doctor or naturalist. Nineteen of them set forth on collecting journeys covering North and South America, Africa, Japan, and the Asian tropics. The worldwide race of exploration was on. Certainly, the primary goals were to gain economic and military power, but knowledge of geology and biology was also a high priority. Navy vessels doubled as scientific labs, and the best collections and collectors were often afloat. Two apostles accompanied Cook on different round-the-world jaunts and several died in faraway places. But the enterprise resulted in an explosion of knowledge about life's diversity. Linnaeus sat in the center of this worldwide web of discovery. His goal was to do for biology what Brahe and Kepler had done for astronomy. The raw data of life, in all its fecund complexity, needed to be sorted into manageable bins. If we could develop a crystallizing classification of all the world's plants and animals, perhaps we could figure out God's design. If gravity is a simple explanation for the seeming complexity of planetary motion, perhaps there is a simple explanation for the diversity of life.

Linnaeus developed a compelling sorting scheme that has survived three hundred years and even manages to accommodate the revolution in modern genetics. He didn't always get the details right, but this really doesn't matter—it was his method that provided the powerful scientific tool. Based on similarities, 7,700 plants and 4,400 animals were sorted, within a six-step nested hierarchy into their appropriate kingdom, phylum, class, order, genus, and species. It worked. Linnaeus brought order to the seemingly chaotic biological universe. In a dramatic departure from previous religious exceptionalism, humans were included within the classification system, right next to apes and monkeys. Though a great blow to our dignity, it was a giant step forward toward the theory of evolution. Linnaeus's careful sorting of descriptive complexity was the necessary precondition for Darwin's simplifying explanation of how life had evolved into all its many niches.

This was the second great demonstration of the three-stage process of observational science. What worked for astronomy also worked for biology. First, you need painstakingly careful descriptions of the natural world. Next, clever classification to reduce the seeming complexity into manageable patterns based on observed similarities. Then finally the payoff—an explanation so simple and obvious that everyone wonders why he or she didn't think of it. It is impossible to come up with right answers until the questions get asked the right way. Any good classification shouts out the question "Why is nature like this?" And the hope is that someone will see causal meaning in the descriptive patterning.

A century later, Mendeleyev got the same ball rolling in physics with his periodic table of the elements. Surprisingly soon, the questions raised by his sorting of the elements led to a deep and simplifying causal model of the different structures of their atomic nuclei. One of the great disappointments of modern medicine and psychiatry is that our classification systems have not succeeded in stimulating clear explanatory models. The body, and especially the brain, have a particularity and complexity that seem to forever deny any easy causal answers.[11]

Philippe Pinel: The Father of Psychiatry

The Renaissance and Enlightenment came late to psychiatry—not until the beginning of the nineteenth century. This is not because the people interested in human behavior were dumber. It is because the topic is so complicated. Planets are a lot simpler and more regular in their motions than brains are in their malfunctions. The general laws of astronomy and biology are much easier to discover than the precise mechanisms causing disease. Modern science wisely picked for initial discovery topics that lent themselves to grand abstractions. Gravity and evolution were remarkable intellectual feats, but they are fairly low-hanging fruit compared to understanding schizophrenia.

Meanwhile the living conditions for the mentally ill had become increasingly dreadful. The Industrial Revolution, population growth, and urbanization had disrupted the old social patterns of management that had mostly been the responsibility of family, village, and priest. The new pressures on working-class families understandably reduced their tolerance and resources for supporting disturbed and disturbing family members. It was more convenient to ship them away to institutional settings often located in faraway places. Patients were confined along with other undesirables—paupers, criminals, orphans, and the intellectually infirm. The often for-profit poorhouses lacked any healing or scientific mission. Mixed in as they were, the mad were seen as bad, their symptoms the result of moral failings and not really of any medical interest. There was no profession of psychiatry and no clinical study that might lead to diagnosis and classification. The mad were considered less than fully human, more like wild animals needing taming, whipping, and chaining, and were subject to zoolike public demonstrations meant to raise revenue.

Philippe Pinel saved the patients and created the profession of psychiatry in the Western world. Our field couldn't possibly have a better father and role model. Both humanist and scientist, he taught us how to treat patients as people—with proper dignity as we study their problems. Pinel is most famous for stripping the chains from the mentally ill. You can still see the marks on the places where they were attached to the wall in an old building on the grounds of the still active psychiatric unit of the Salpêtrière Hospital in Paris. But Pinel gave them a bigger gift. He stripped away the medieval superstition that mental illness was demon possession and that its victims were to be dreaded, denigrated, neglected, perhaps even burned at the stake. He convinced (almost) everyone that mental illness comes from entirely natural causes equivalent to the causes of medical illness. And he developed a new model of "asylum" care devoted exclusively to the needs of the mentally ill, who he felt should be treated with respect in a pleasant and safe environment. Soon similar "asylum" hospitals sprang up all over Europe and the United States.

Pinel liked his patients as people and treated them as if they were simply human. When given the choice of joining Napoléon as personal physician or staying with his patients, he turned down Napoléon. Pinel's chief administrator, advisor, and teacher was a former inmate who had become a brilliant clinician and manager. Together they developed a "moral" (or "psychological") treatment for mental illness that combined education, cognitive therapy, reality testing, work, exercise, therapeutic activities, support, and encouragement—all delivered with kindness, modesty, and a sense of humor. Pinel was deeply interested in each patient's life story—the particular hopes, fears, motives, and circumstances that shape who we are. He wanted to learn how their troubles in life interacted with the illness.

Pinel believed mental disease was caused by some combination of heredity, physiological damage to the brain, psychological and social stress, and the previous hideous treatment the patients had often received. He wanted to facilitate a natural healing, not a forced cure. No more bleeding, purging, blistering, or spin chairs. He was modest about what he could accomplish and trusted the resilience and healing powers of his patients. Physical restraint with a straitjacket and chemical restraint with opium were reserved only for those who were most violent and responded to nothing else.

Beyond being a wonderful person, Pinel was also a good scientist. He combined the syndrome approach of Sydenham and the classifying methods of Linnaeus to sort the symptoms of mental illness into convenient categories. The diagnostic labels used in psychiatry would be based on a natural science approach of minute observation. He spent a great deal of time with his patients, questioning in detail to determine the most frequent clustering of symptoms and the evolution of their course. His suggested categories were somewhat different from those used today, but our current methods of classification are the ones he introduced. As in everything, Pinel was modest. He presented his suggestions tentatively, "for the time being."

Pinel begins modern psychiatry and ends its dark ages. The growth of psychiatry in the nineteenth century made the classification of mental disorders an exciting endeavor on both humane and intellectual grounds. Beyond the obvious clinical purpose, there was the notion that clearly describing and demarcating the mental disorders might lead to better theories of what caused them. The classifiers were clinicians, but they were also observational scientists, doing for psychiatric diagnosis what Linnaeus had done for plants and animals. If they did a good enough job of describing, perhaps a psychiatric Darwin would come along and make sense of it all.[12]

Following Pinel, there was an amazing flurry of creative classifying—a succession of different ways of sorting psychiatric disorders was suggested during the remaining years of the nineteenth century. The early systems were French, but then the center of scientific gravity gradually shifted to Germany, culminating in Emil Kraepelin's crucial distinction between schizophrenia and bipolar disorder. It was a lucky coincidence that Kraepelin's brother was a great naturalist—this sharpened his own considerable observational skills and also forced him to find ways to raise funds to support their frequent joint field trips to East Asia. Kraepelin's moonlighting job changed the history of psychiatry. The table of contents of his remarkably popular and influential textbook became the *DSM* of its time and later formed the basis for our own *DSM*s. But Kraepelin had a big blind spot—he was a hospital-based doctor who never saw an outpatient. His conception of psychiatry was formed by, and restricted to, those who were ill enough to require long-term confinement, and his classification lacked appropriate niches for most of the people who are diagnosed today.

Lucky again that Freud happened to be around to fill this gap. People usually associate Freud with treatment, not diagnosis—but he did as much to figure out the classification of the outpatient conditions as Kraepelin had done for the inpatient. Interestingly, Freud had also become a classifier only because he too was very short on cash, in his case to get married and start a family. Early in his career, Freud had been a very promising neuroscientist, one of the pioneers in understanding the importance of the neuronal synapse in brain functioning. But unable to land a university job, he was forced out of the laboratory and into the less exalted private practice of neurology. Accepting this career reversal with considerable regret and reluctance, Freud never abandoned his original ambition to achieve scientific recognition. Instead he switched his object of investigation from slides to people. Soon he became the Darwin of the consulting room, using astute clinical observations to make strikingly accurate guesses on how unconscious, inborn instincts play a central role in who we are, what we feel, how we think, and what we do—both in sickness and in health. Modern cognitive science and brain imaging have provided convincing confirmation of Freud's most profound insights—even if some of his other guesses now seem quaintly off the wall.

More pertinent here, Freud also opened up the new profession of outpatient psychiatry and provided it with a way of classifying its new patients. The milder symptom presentations that are now the bread and butter of psychiatry were then the province of neurologists, who had named them "neuroses" in the belief they were caused by nerve disease. In developing the altogether new field of psychoanalysis, Freud reconceptualized "neurosis" as being due to psychological conflict—conditioned by the biology of the brain, but not a simple brain disease. And then he proceeded to classify the neuroses—separating mourning from melancholia; panic disorder from phobias and generalized anxiety; and describing obsessive-compulsive disorder, the sexual disorders, and the personality disorders. Freud was a trained neurologist who had spent only a few months studying psychiatry. Paradoxically, he was largely ignored by the neurologists but soon came to be very much adored by the psychiatrists.

The early psychiatrists were few in number, worked exclusively in inpatient asylums, and were burdened with the unfortunate title "alienists." But following Freud, this all changed and changed quickly. The specialty of psychiatry switched its focus from very sick inpatients to not-so-sick outpatients. Psychiatrists left hospitals in droves to establish outpatient office practices; whereas in 1917, only 10 percent of psychiatrists practiced outside hospitals, now most do.[13] The numbers of psychoanalysts inside the United States were also swelled by prominent refugees who were fleeing the Nazis and by mental health clinicians from the burgeoning new professions of psychology and social work. A quickly expanding group of therapists was treating a much larger, but also much less ill, outpatient population, using the new set of milder outpatient diagnoses derived from psychoanalysis.

Simultaneously, the world wars were broadening the boundaries of psychiatry and bringing it into the mainstream. Psychiatric illness was identified as a major threat to the war effort—a frequent cause of unfitness for duty; a common form of combat casualty; and a source of continuing disability in those who returned home. Existing classifications, designed for severely ill hospitalized inpatients, were not up to the task of diagnosing what ailed the troops. Psychiatrists were called in to refine the system and figure out how to keep our soldiers ready for combat. Many rose to high military rank (including one general) and had extraordinary influence in decisions regarding recruitment, retention, and combat treatment.[14] A new and expanded diagnostic classification was devised by the army, revised by the Veterans Administration and revised again by the American Psychiatric Association as the *Diagnostic and Statistical Manual I,* published in 1952.[15]

DSM-III Saves Psychiatry

Psychiatry blossomed after World War II—having proven its wartime mettle, it gained a newly prominent role in civilian life. Separate psychiatry departments were created for the first time at all the medical schools, and new psychiatric units were opened in most general hospitals. The predominant model was psychoanalytic; the focus was on treatment; and the attitude was can-do professional confidence. Meanwhile, psychiatric diagnosis enjoyed none of this renaissance—it was a quiet and insignificant backwater completely ignored in all the excitement. *DSM-I* (published in 1952) and *DSM-II* (published in 1968) were unread, unloved, and unused.[16, 17]

Then suddenly, in the early 1970s, diagnosis was exposed as the Achilles' heel that might bring psychiatry down. Two widely publicized papers posed an existential threat to its recently acquired credential as a full-fledged medical specialty. First shocker: a cross-national British/American study found that psychiatrists on the different sides of the pond differed radically in their diagnostic conclusions, even when evaluating the same patients on videotape.[18] Second shocker: a clever psychologist showed how easy it was to lure psychiatrists into providing not only inaccurate diagnoses but also wildly inappropriate treatment. Several of his graduate students went to different emergency rooms stating they were hearing voices. Every single one was promptly admitted to a psychiatric hospital despite thereafter acting in a perfectly normal manner, and each was kept for several weeks to several months. Psychiatrists looked like unreliable and antiquated quacks, unfit to join in the research revolution just then about to modernize the rest of medicine.

Without Robert Spitzer, psychiatry might have become increasingly irrelevant, drifting back to its prewar obscurity. It is rare that one man saves a profession, but psychiatry badly needed saving, and Bob was a rare man. Then a young researcher at Columbia University, he had already embarked on what was to become an almost fanatic, lifelong quest to make psychiatric diagnosis systematic and reliable. Think Ahab relentlessly chasing Moby Dick.

Bob had been among the pioneers in creating the checklists of the Research Diagnostic Criteria—a criteria-based method of sorting symptoms into disorders that increased the diagnostic agreement of raters participating in research studies.[19] He had also developed semistructured interview instruments that controlled the vagaries of evaluation by suggesting a uniform sequence and wording of the questions used to assess the presence or absence of each symptom.[20] Early findings using Bob's methods were encouraging—raters achieved reasonably good agreement if they asked the same questions and used the same rules of the road in going from symptom counts to diagnosis. This met the challenge posed by the cross-national study. More important, a reliable diagnostic system provided psychiatric research with the means to employ the incredible new tools of molecular biology, genetics, brain imaging, multivariate statistics, and placebo-controlled clinical trials. Suddenly research in psychiatry became a darling, no longer the stepchild, of medical research. The budget of the National Institute of Mental Health grew rapidly, and in most medical schools, psychiatry became the second biggest source of research funding—just after the department of internal medicine and far ahead of all the other basic science and clinical departments. Drug companies also began pouring in loads of research money as they raced to develop profitable new psychiatric medicines.

Spitzer had laid the foundations for the psychiatric research enterprise. Many people might have been content, but Bob was a man of restless spirit and soon realized that there were much bigger fish to fry. If the criteria-based method of diagnosis worked so well in research studies, why not also apply it to everyday clinical practice? This was an outrageously audacious ambition, but the American Psychiatric Association offered Bob the perfect opportunity to realize it. In 1975, he was asked to chair the *DSM-III* Task Force and given wide authority to set his own goals, choose methods, and pick collaborators. Spitzer was energetic, determined, stubborn, and indomitable—an enthusiastic true believer in whatever he was doing. His goal was nothing less than to transform psychiatric practice as performed everywhere in the world and by all the mental health disciplines. As Bob himself put it at the time, "They gave me the ball and I ran with it." *DSM-III* [21] would end the diagnostic anarchy, would focus attention on careful diagnosis as a necessary prerequisite to more precise and specific treatment selection, and would also form a much-needed bridge between clinical research and clinical psychiatry.[22]

The development of *DSM-III* faced one great handicap. There was very limited scientific evidence then available to guide any of its decisions—that is, which disorders should be included in the manual and which symptoms should be chosen to describe each disorder. Bob filled the huge gaps by bringing together small groups of experts on each disorder and picking their brains to thrash out how best to define the criteria sets.

The process wasn't pretty to watch—it had the feel more of virtuoso performance art than scientific deliberation. The meetings all followed a remarkably uniform pattern. A group of about eight or ten experts would be virtually locked down in a room and were not to emerge until they could come to an agreement. The mornings were loud and unruly—with experts shouting out what they thought were the best symptoms, often disagreeing vociferously with one another. Their passionate views were argued with the fierce determination that comes from lived experience, rather than scientific data, and there seemed to be no rational way of choosing among their differing suggestions. Bob would be mostly quiet—typing fast and furiously in a corner, trying to get it all down. After a few anarchic hours, a big tray of terrific deli food would arrive. The experts would finally quiet down as they instead worked over the sandwiches, slaw, pickles, and cream soda. Bob would keep typing furiously, totally focused and seemingly oblivious to the food or his surroundings. Miraculously, by lunch's end, Bob would have digested the morning's chaos into a draft criteria set that neatly condensed into one coherent definition all the divergent suggestions. The afternoon would usually be much calmer, the drowsy experts fine-tuning Bob's compromise product. Whenever controversy did persist, the advantage went to whoever was most loud, confident, stubborn, senior, or spoke to Bob last. This is a terrible way to develop a diagnostic system, which would be subject to all sorts of biases, but it was the best way available at the time. And the surprise is that it worked as well as it did. The product was surely flawed but also remarkably useful.

Bob's colleagues in developing these criteria sets were mostly the young Turks of psychiatry (and a few psychologists)—the newly emerging and closely knit cohort of biologically oriented researchers who saw themselves as a vanguard pushing the field toward the rest of medicine and away from the previously dominant psychoanalytic and social models. *DSM-III* was advertised as atheoretical in regard to etiology and equally applicable to the biological, psychological, and social models of treatment. This was true on paper but not in fact. It was true in that the criteria sets were based on surface symptoms and said nothing about causes or treatments. But the surface symptoms method fit very neatly with a biological, medical model of mental disorder and greatly promoted it. The rejection of more inferential psychological constructs and social context severely disadvantaged these other models and put psychiatry into something of a reductionistic straitjacket. *DSM-III* tried to make up for this by introducing an innovative "multiaxial" system—patients were rated not just on Axis I psychiatric symptoms but also on Axis II personality disorders, Axis III medical illness, Axis IV social stressors, and Axis V, overall level of functioning. Unfortunately, the multiaxial system was mostly ignored. For a time Bob proposed a "let a hundred flowers bloom" project that would have highlighted all the factors beyond descriptive diagnosis that should contribute to a complete evaluation—but this never got off the ground. Proponents of psychological or social models felt left out of the game and have steadily lost status and influence since the publication of *DSM-III*.

Revolutions are never easy or complete. Bob was an irresistible force wrestling with hundreds of thousands of seemingly immovable objects. Clinicians in those days hated to be herded (they have since been mostly tamed). *DSM-III* lumped patients based on surface similarities, ignoring their individual differences. In contrast, psychologically minded clinicians preferred to rely on empathy and creative intuition to understand each patient's complex life story, unconscious motivations, and social context. They didn't want to be boxed in, mindlessly following rote rules imposed impersonally from without. The simpleminded *DSM-III* approach was absolutely necessary if psychiatrists were to agree on diagnosis—but it seemed to leave out almost everything that was most interesting about the patient. Bob was providing a lingua franca, but not one that was very attractive to most of the people who would have to use it. He was turning the poetry of individual patients into *DSM-III* prose.

I started out a strong *DSM-III* skeptic and was a late and only partial convert.

Bob and I went back ten years before *DSM-III*. He had been a teacher of mine in the late 1960s—someone I liked very much personally but had largely discounted professionally because he focused all his attention on what I thought were superficial and dumb diagnostic questions. What I cared about then was learning what motivations made people tick and how I could help them get on a bit better in life through psychotherapy. When a few years later, Bob began working on *DSM-III*, I was slightly older, not much wiser, and not the least bit interested. My job then was running the outpatient department at Cornell–New York Hospital; my expensive hobby was completing psychoanalytic training at Columbia, where I would occasionally run into Bob in the hallways. During one of our brief chats, I made what now seems a screwball suggestion—that *DSM-III* include a masochistic personality disorder to describe people who, for unconscious masochistic reasons, repetitively sabotage their opportunities for happiness in life. This was an idea I was studying in class and thinking about as a possible topic for a psychoanalytic paper. Bob rightly nixed it, just as I did later when someone else suggested it for *DSM-IV*. He explained that it was far too inferential to ever be assessed reliably and that all psychiatric disorder is inherently self-defeating. But Bob's approach was ecumenical, and he would instinctively recruit to the *DSM-III* team anyone willing to spend time feeding his voracious and insatiable appetite for diagnostic discussion. Soon I was busily at work on *DSM-III*, assigned the tasks of editing the personality disorders section and also of explaining and justifying the new *DSM-III* methods to my skeptical colleagues in the several different psychoanalytic associations.

As I gradually came to know *DSM-III* really well, I could much better appreciate its necessity, but also better understand its inherent limitations. My impression then, which still feels right now, is that

DSM-III was absolutely essential but also greatly oversold and over-bought. It was the salvation of a scientifically based psychiatry but also truncated the purview of the field and triggered harmful diagnostic inflation. *DSM-III* was essential because it brought system to the diagnosis and treatment of mental disorders. Previously psychiatry was pure art form—sometimes brilliant, usually idiosyncratic, and always chaotic. There still remains much that is usefully artful in psychiatry, but now there is standardization and a firmer scientific foundation.

But the much-trumpeted reliability of *DSM-III* was oversold because the level of diagnostic agreement obtained under ideal circumstances in research settings can never be achieved in the rough-and-tumble of average clinical practice. *DSM-III* was also wildly overbought—both literally and metaphorically. To everyone's surprise, it became a perennial best seller with hundreds of thousands of copies sold every year, many more than there are mental health workers. *DSM-III* was the victim of its own success—it became the "bible" of psychiatry to the exclusion of other aspects of the field that should not have been, but were, cast beneath its shadow. Diagnosis should just be one part of a complete evaluation, but instead it became dominant. Understanding the whole patient was often reduced to filling out a checklist. Lost in the shuffle were the narrative arc of the patient's life and the contextual factors influencing symptom formation. This was not an inherent flaw of *DSM-III*—rather it came from *DSM-III* being given far too much authority by clinicians, teachers and their students, researchers, insurance companies, school systems, disability agencies, and the courts. And by the public. *DSM-III* diagnosis quickly replaced psychoanalysis as a topic of cocktail party chatter, and people seemed eager to find a neat fit for their problems (or their boss's problems) in its pages.

Diagnostic inflation has been the worst consequence of *DSM-III*. Part of the fault lies in how *DSM-III* was written, much of it in how it has been misused, particularly under the influence of drug company disease mongering. *DSM-III* was a splitter's dream and a lumper's nightmare—and splitting inherently leads to diagnostic inflation. To increase the likelihood that clinicians would agree on a given diagnosis, *DSM-III* divided the diagnostic pie into many very small and easily digested slices—but this also increased the likelihood that many more people would be diagnosed. Add to this that *DSM-III* was also overly inclusive—with many new mental disorders describing mild symptom presentations at the populous boundary with normality. The fact that *DSM-III* was suddenly so interesting to clinicians and patients also stimulated more diagnosing.

Given the conditions in 1980 when it was published, *DSM-III* probably struck a pretty fair balance between sensitivity (its errors in missing people who needed a diagnosis) and specificity (its errors in mislabeling people who didn't need diagnosis). At the time, no one understood that this seesaw would soon be weighed down so heavily on the side of overdiagnosis. The seeds of diagnostic inflation that had been planted by *DSM-III* would soon become giant beanstalks when nourished by drug company marketing.

DSM-IIIR—Too Much, Too Soon

DSM-IIIR was the revision of *DSM-III* published just seven years later in 1987. It was meant to be a small makeover, no more than a minor midterm correction of the errors and omissions noted after the publication of *DSM-III*. Bob Spitzer was in charge again, and this time his enormous energy and enthusiasm got out of hand. The project went on twice as long as originally scheduled and made many major changes—all in the direction of making it easier to get a psychiatric diagnosis. I was part of the inner circle advising Bob on *DSM-IIIR*,[23] but his eagerness for change and enthusiasm for expansion were impossible to contain.

DSM-IIIR was a mistake and a distraction. One goal of *DSM-III* was to create a kind of Linnaean classification (or "periodic table") of objectively defined mental disorders that would then stimulate clinical and basic science research. The system was meant to be iterative and self-correcting—taking what were essentially the made-up criteria sets in *DSM-III* as the starting point, but then confirming or altering them based on the research they promoted. This circular process could never proceed if the diagnostic system offered a moving research target, constantly shifting capriciously, based on arbitrary opinion.

The lesson for me was that diagnosis needed to rest in order to let research catch up. It made no sense to keep rearranging the furniture of descriptive psychiatry, creating new diagnoses or altering the thresholds of existing ones, based only on the whims of the experts who happened to be in the room. The method that was necessary for *DSM-III* had been inappropriate for *DSM-IIIR*. Changes in diagnoses should be few and far between until we gained a much deeper understanding of what causes the mental disorders and how best to define and treat them. *DSM-III* had of necessity come mostly out of the heads of the experts as translated into "manualese" by Bob Spitzer. The future required more caution, tighter scientific standards, less personal opinion, and no change just for change's sake.

The full reality of diagnostic inflation was years away, but the threat was in the air. Prozac and *DSM-IIIR* were both introduced in 1987. Prozac's sales took off at least in part because the *DSM* definition of major depressive disorder was so loose. The message was clear—psychotropic drugs offered vast market potential, and sales could be greatly influenced by *DSM* decisions. It was important that the diagnostic system not become an unwitting tool of drug company marketing.

The *DSM-IV* Story

When asked why I was picked to head the *DSM-IV* Task Force, I usually joke it was a punishment inflicted for sins in a prior life. The serious point is that I don't really know why I was picked and the process was remarkably casual. The medical director of the American Psychiatric Association asked if I would accept the appointment. I thought about it for a day and said yes. Simple as that. No muss, no fuss, no vetting, no interviews, no competition, no testing of my qualifications, goals, or methods.

By illustrative contrast, the selection marathon that preceded my appointment as chair of psychiatry at Duke University took four months and included: three search committee meetings; numerous conversations with the dean; meetings with the head of the hospital, the president of the university, the financial officer, the chairs of all the other departments, and with about fifty members of the department. Even before all this, a representative of the search committee had called at least thirty people to check me out. Before hiring me, Duke knew more about me than I knew about myself. The careful vetting process guaranteed that we would have a jointly worked-out agenda and plan of action.

In contrast, the APA took me mostly on faith, with little idea how I would proceed. They probably chose me because I had worked on the two previous *DSM*s and was chair of the APA Committee on Diagnosis; to that degree, I was a known quantity. And there weren't that many people who had the background to do the job or would be willing to. But a formal search would have ensured I was the best choice and would have made my plans and the charge much clearer. The casual selection process left me with far too much discretion.

There was also almost no direction from APA on picking the colleagues who would work with me on *DSM-IV* and how to proceed in preparing it. The natural tendency is to recruit your friends. It will be more fun working with people you like and much easier to lean on them to put in the many unpaid hours needed to get the job done. I decided instead to include all the opposing views on what I anticipated would be the most controversial questions. But no one made me do this.

We set goals for *DSM-IV* that were extremely modest—to introduce rigor, objectivity, and transparency in how decisions were made, and not to innovate or add personal touches to the system.[24, 25] I knew that if we set a high scientific burden of proof, few changes would be made because there would not be convincing evidence to support them. Data rarely jump off the page, grab you by the throat, and insist you make a change. The strange thing is that APA had so little idea what my goals would be and so little input in shaping the direction of *DSM-IV*. This was a mistake. No single person should be left free to determine the future of a diagnostic system that has such wide influence. The numerous problems that afflicted *DSM-5* illustrate the risks inherent to unchecked, potentially idiosyncratic leadership.

Which brings up the question of leadership style. I was following in the footsteps of a charismatic leader who took a passionate interest in each and every question and loved the controversies that surrounded them. Bob's approach was appropriate to the task of creating out of whole cloth a radically new diagnostic system, but creativity and innovation were not the skills best suited to the minor course corrections required for *DSM-IIIR* or *DSM-IV*. The seven years each between *DSM-III*, *DSM-IIIR*, and *DSM-IV* (1980, 1987, and 1994) hadn't generated compelling research findings to warrant a significant revision of the diagnostic system. I therefore saw my role as one of refiner/conservator rather than innovator. Requiring a high level of scientific proof before any change took most of the personality and leadership issues out of the equation. I set up an impersonal system that would work automatically to avoid and solve controversies. Decision making was to follow rules rather than clashing personal convictions. The role of work group member was defined as "consensus scholar" quietly reviewing tables of available data, not advocating for a cause or aspiring to be an innovative diagnostic pathfinder.

I don't like controversies and find them unproductive—almost all heat, very rarely any light. So we took the realistic position that any prolonged disagreements on the interpretation of data meant the scientific literature was too sparse or ambiguous to support change. A change would be made only when it was compellingly necessary and there was an overwhelming consensus on the science. This didn't happen very often. Anything close to a hung jury was decided in favor of the status quo. There were no votes, and I don't remember any serious disagreements.

Having hundreds of strong-minded experts working on a project could be a recipe for anarchy. The antidote was to set up standard operating procedures and to make sure that everyone followed them closely. All of the timelines for doing *DSM-IV* were established well before we began work on it. A series of methods conferences ensured that every procedure would be performed in a consistent way. The threshold for making changes was clear, uniform, and rigorous. We established a three-stage obstacle course intended to weed out new suggestions. Stage 1 was a searching literature review that would painstakingly gather the available scientific data, with special consideration given to the possible risks and unintended consequences of any change. Stage 2 consisted of data reanalyses funded by the MacArthur Foundation. This allowed us to access already collected but not yet analyzed data sets that lived in the computers of investigators around the world. We could ask questions pertaining to *DSM-IV* decisions that had not yet been answered in the published literature. Stage 3 consisted of NIMH-funded, peer-reviewed field trials covering twelve disorders where changes were contemplated. The goal was to test-drive the alternative criteria sets to see how they compared under conditions that approximated (but did not duplicate) real life.

The role of the central leadership was quality control. Our job was not to decide issues, but rather to ensure that the rules were followed. It was also our job to guarantee that all deadlines would be met. The result of all this methodological rigor was exactly what we expected. The pet proposals of the experts were consistently shot down because the science wasn't there to support them. *DSM-IV* was faithful to *DSM-IIIR*.

All our work was a completely open book with extremely porous boundaries. Anyone showing interest in *DSM-IV* could become an advisor to the process. Work group members were encouraged to tell all and get full input from colleagues. At midpoint an Options Book was published that gave everyone a chance to vet and shoot down all proposed changes. We also published an extensive four-volume *DSM-IV* Sourcebook as an archival resource, including all of the literature reviews, data reanalyses, field trials, and rationales for decisions.[26] As we shall see, *DSM-5* went far wrong in large part because it was secretive and closed to outside correction.

We saw *DSM-IV* as a guidebook, not a bible—a collection of temporarily useful diagnostic constructs, not a catalog of "real" diseases. We tried to make this abundantly clear in the introduction to *DSM-IV* and at greater length in the *DSM-IV* Guidebook. Unfortunately, I am not sure anyone ever reads the introduction, and I know that few people have read the Guidebook.[27, 28] People shouldn't worship the *DSM* categories, but it does make you a better clinician to know them.

DSM-IV did not save normal, or even protect it very well. Three years after its publication, drug company lobbyists won a huge victory over sensible regulation. The United States became the only country in the world that allows direct-to-consumer advertising of pharmaceuticals. Pretty soon the airwaves and print were filled with glowingly misleading representations that everyday problems were in fact unrecognized psychiatric disorder. *DSM-IV* turned out to be a very weak dike unable to block the flood of false demand instigated by the aggressive and devilishly clever drug company push. Although we had consistently rejected suggestions that would have benefited drug companies, we failed to predict that even our conservative manual could provide such easy fodder for advertising gold. Within a few years, it was clear the drug companies had won and we had lost.

There were steps we could (and probably should) have taken to help curb diagnostic inflation. Most important, we could have tightened the *DSM-IV* diagnostic thresholds (required more symptoms, longer durations, and greater impairment) to make it more difficult for companies to sell diagnoses. But we had hoisted ourselves on our own perhaps too evenhanded, conservative petard—our strict evidentiary rules required the presence of extensive and compelling scientific data before we could make any change in either direction. Following our rules made it just as difficult to deflate the diagnostic system as to inflate it. The rules were a necessary constraint to contain arbitrary decision making and the experts' natural tendencies to expand their own domains. Being evidence-based rather than opinion-driven helped us avoid contributing to new inflation, but it also prevented us from reducing the inflation that was already in place. Knowing what I know now, this was probably a mistake. It would have been better to create a double standard, with less evidence required to effect deflation than to promote inflation. Admittedly, deflation would have been difficult and arbitrary, but it now seems preferable to the excessive diagnosis and treatment that have since been protected by our adherence to evidence.

And there was much more we could have done to sound warnings. We should have been far more active in educating the field and prospective patients about the risks of overdiagnosis. There should have been prominent cautions in *DSM-IV* warning about overdiagnosis and providing tips on how to avoid it. We should have organized professional and public conferences and educational campaigns to counteract drug company propaganda. None of this occurred to anyone at the time. No one dreamed that drug company advertising would explode three years after the publication of *DSM-IV* or that there would be the huge epidemics of ADHD, autism, and bipolar disorder—and therefore no one felt any urgency to prevent them. We thought we had done a reasonably good job of writing the manual and didn't see it as our responsibility to make sure it was used responsibly. We missed the boat. Even if we had been smarter and tougher we probably couldn't have stemmed the tide of overdiagnosis. Big Pharma was simply too big, too rich, and too politically powerful. But I do very much regret that we didn't try harder.

So what is my final scorecard on *DSM-IV*? Decidedly mixed. On the positive side: We made very few changes; developed and implemented a meticulous method of scientific review; improved the precision of the manual's writing and coding; and made only one obvious mistake. On the negative side: Our changes contributed directly to the false epidemics of autistic, attention deficit, and adult bipolar disorder; we did nothing to prevent the overdiagnosis of several other disorders that have been puffed up by the drug companies; and our one outright mistake was a disaster, a sloppily worded paraphilia section that has allowed the widespread unconstitutional abuse of involuntary psychiatric hospitalization. We could have done a lot worse, but we should have done better in predicting unintended consequences and preventing continued diagnostic inflation. Trying hard to be rigorous and "do no harm" protected us from most errors of commission but forced us into serious errors of omission. We didn't do much harm, but we weren't of much help. When it was completed, I was pretty happy with *DSM-IV*. Now I wish we had done more to save normal and reduce the ease with which the drug companies were able to sell sickness.

A legitimate question has been raised about the motivations of the people working on *DSM-IV*—did we go soft on diagnostic inflation because of a financial conflict of interest? The concern arises from a recent study showing that 56 percent of our experts had some financial connection to drug companies. The assertion has been made that the companies were pulling strings behind the scenes, directly or subtly, to bend decisions toward more diagnosis and more treatment. The question is certainly legitimate because we had no formal conflict of interest policy or vetting system. This omission was a silly mistake on our part—the necessity simply never occurred to any of us when we began work in the fairly innocent pre-Prozac days of 1987. There is no excuse for our failure to put in place the formal tools of protection against conflict of interest. I apologize for this but don't agree that financial conflict of interest compromised any of our decisions. The proof is in the pudding. The results prove that our rigorous method of review successfully protected against any potential conflict of interest just as surely as the most thorough vetting ever could. Dozens of proposals that would have favored drug companies were shot down. Only two of our decisions wound up helping drug companies—slightly loosening the requirements for attention deficit disorder and introducing bipolar II. Both of these filled an important clinical niche, both were supported by substantial evidence, and neither had much obvious commercial value when the decisions were made. Unfortunately, both decisions were later exploited by the drug companies when they gained the right to advertise to consumers and had developed new and expensive products to sell—but this happened in ways we could not have predicted or prevented. The drug industry played no role whatever in how *DSM-IV* was written, but played the deciding role in how it was misused. I agree that Caesar's wife should be above suspicion—but also feel certain that in this case the suspicion is misplaced.[29,30]

The *DSMs* have a mixed record. They have served an extremely valuable function in improving the reliability of psychiatric diagnosis and in encouraging a revolution in psychiatric research. But they have also had the very harmful unintended consequence of triggering and helping to maintain a runaway diagnostic inflation that threatens normal and results in massive overtreatment with psychiatric medication.

CHAPTER 3

Diagnostic Inflation

Alice: "But I don't want to go among mad people."
Cheshire Cat: "Oh, you can't help it, we're all mad here."
LEWIS CARROLL, *Alice's Adventures in Wonderland*

Medical research has made such enormous advances that
there are hardly any healthy people left.
ALDOUS HUXLEY

DIAGNOSTIC INFLATION HAS many, many causes and will require many cures. Some of the problems are inherent to psychiatry and need curing from within the profession. But a number of powerful outside forces flexed their muscles, grabbed hold of *DSM-IV*, and used clever methods to encourage its misuse. They succeeded in changing diagnostic habits in ways we never imagined possible and lacked the tools to control. The past thirty years have witnessed a frightening vicious cycle. Diagnostic inflation has led to an explosive growth in the use of psychotropic drugs; this then produced huge profits that have given the pharmaceutical industry the means and the motive to blow up the diagnostic bubble into an ever-expanding balloon. The coinage of psychiatric diagnosis has been cheapened, making "normal" a scarce commodity. Just as happens with monetary inflation, the bad money drives the good out of circulation and resources allocation is distorted. The wasted effort devoted to those who don't have real disorders deprives those who do from receiving badly needed psychiatric diagnosis and care.

Causes of Diagnostic Inflation

Following the Pied Piper of Diagnostic Inflation in the Rest of Medicine

Psychiatry didn't invent diagnostic inflation—it has just blindly followed the crowd in turning seeming wellness into dreaded sickness. The rest of medicine got there first by promoting the idea that all of us need to have regularly repeated batteries of screening tests to find out what might be going wrong with our bodies, even before we are experiencing any symptoms of illness. What an appealing goal—screen early to prevent disease before it can gain traction and cause harm. Not only would this reduce human suffering, but it would also save money. Detect cancer before it can spread; treat the slightest increase in blood pressure before it causes heart disease; control blood sugar before it becomes full-fledged diabetes; stop bone loss before osteoporosis causes fractures. At its most telling extreme, people subjected themselves to yearly full-body CAT scans to clearly visualize every internal nook and cranny—until it became clear that the test was worse than the disease. The risks of getting cancer from the X-ray exposure far outweighed any potential benefit in picking up early cancers. Preventive intervention would be wonderful, if only we had an accurate way to identify who needs it. But most early screening picks up lots of people who are better left alone.[1]

The hype for prevention has been everywhere. Breakthroughs in medical science are breathlessly announced daily. New tests are constantly being devised and the thresholds of abnormality of old tests lowered—creating hordes of new patients. Doctors order expensive batteries of every conceivable test on every patient, just to be on the safe side. Advertisements promote the benefits of screening and the terrors of letting disease go unfettered. The screening scare tactics have been an enormous financial success for their promoters, but the evidence shows that with few exceptions (e.g., screening for lung cancer in smokers or colon cancer in everyone), the testing is often not good for the patients—not really improving outcomes, while further burdening them with aggressive, expensive, and unnecessary treatments. And the waste to society runs to hundreds of billions of dollars a year that could be better used treating really sick people who are currently not insured. [Preventive medicine is a terrific goal gone badly astray because it became industrialized and enslaved by profit and hype.]

Sanity is beginning to prevail. Recently, nine professional societies have initiated a "Choosing Wisely" campaign, publishing a list of forty-five previously heralded tests and procedures that had been vastly oversold.[2] Prostate cancer screening is no longer recommended—it failed to save lives and resulted in much needlessly aggressive surgery. Breast cancer screening has been much truncated. No more CT scans for headaches or X-rays for back pain. And it turns out that bronchodilators and oxygen don't work for most people with chronic obstructive pulmonary disease.[3] The list is long and telling. Evidence-based medicine is demonstrating that the push to prevention has been excessive, premature, and not evidence based.

Early identification of illness suffers from the "needle in the haystack" problem. Screening tests routinely set their bar low so as not to miss people who need identifying but in the process inevitably wind up mislabeling lots of people who don't.[4,5] The benefits to the few, if any, are outweighed by the harms to the many. Some of the misleading hype for early intervention comes from the good faith enthusiasm of medical researchers and practitioners eager to help patients fight disease. But best advice for them comes from the White Rabbit in Alice in Wonderland: "Don't just do something, stand there."

And the profit motive also plays a part. Fifty years ago, President Eisenhower presciently predicted the economic and social damage that would be caused by a too-powerful military-industrial complex.[6] In a parallel development, we have witnessed the explosive growth of a too-powerful medical-industrial complex comprising Big Pharma, insurance companies, testing laboratories, equipment and device makers, hospitals, and doctors—all eager to expand the market by creating a new reservoir of allegedly "about-to-be-sick" well people who need testing and treatment to avoid ever becoming sick in the future.

The United States spends almost twice as much on per capita medical care as the rest of the world.[7] This is a terrific drain on our economy and our $2 trillion investment has paltry returns. We get mediocre medical outcomes, excessively test and treat those without need, and fail to provide adequate care for many in great need. You probably couldn't design a less efficient or less equitable system if you tried hard to do so.

Meanwhile we neglect what are the best forms of prevention—i.e., promoting exercise, proper diet, moderation in alcohol use, abstention from tobacco and drugs. These extremely useful and remarkably cheap prevention measures aren't profitable for the medical-industrial complex and therefore lack its powerful and well-financed sponsorship. The biggest improvement in the health of our country in the last thirty-five years came from the relatively inexpensive campaign to reduce smoking—not from the enormously expensive efforts of the medical-industrial complex. A similar campaign to reduce overtesting and overtreatment would save us money and make us healthier. Let's hope that "choosing wisely" helps to correct the excesses of preventive medicine.

And let's hope that the snake oil of premature preventive medicine doesn't spread to psychiatry. Those who promote the value of wider boundaries for psychiatric disorder make the argument that identifying and treating the mildly mentally ill will help them avoid later becoming the severely mentally ill, drawing support from the presumed glowing success that has been achieved by medical screening and early intervention.[8] But there is a serious fly in this ointment— early intervention in medicine is mostly a flop and provides a terrible model. Psychiatry is wrongheadedly copycatting the very worst aspects of American medicine—the combination of harmful excess for some, combined with heartless neglect for others.

Is Our Stressful Society Making Us Sicker?

One theory says that rates of mental illness are rising because we live under extreme pressures from a speeded-up, stressful society. Perhaps it is hard to be normal because our modern world is driving us crazy. This suggestion is difficult to disprove, but I find it completely unconvincing. Among the hundreds of thousands of generations of our ancestors who have ever walked this earth, we are undoubtedly the luckiest— extraordinarily privileged to live now and to live here. Previous generations (as well as people currently living in less favored parts of our crowded globe) suffer daily catastrophes that are unimaginable to most of us. Life has always been, and will always be, enormously stressful in one or another way. Indeed, our mental discomforts can preoccupy us as much as they do only because most of us don't have to worry about our next meal or the threat of being eaten by a passing tiger.

A second variant of the toxic environment hypothesis is that rates of mental illness have been driven up by physical, rather than emotional, stresses. The most popular version of this is the completely discredited, but ever lingering, belief that vaccination causes autism.[9] Other environmental causes seem equally implausible—fluctuations in diagnostic rates follow a time course much more consonant with fashion than with toxin.

The only environmental pollutants to have a proven substantial impact on mental disorder are alcohol and drugs. These hit the brain with a huge wallop that can mimic virtually all the psychiatric symptoms in the book. But alcohol and drugs can account for only a small part of diagnostic inflation. Tellingly, it is the childhood disorders not much affected by substances that have recently expanded the most.[10]

A third theory has it that we are not sicker than before, just better able to spot previously missed sickness. Some part of diagnostic inflation is surely desirable—picking up previously missed cases. But only a part, and probably a small one. Diagnostic labels can't be applied with surgical precision to accurately distinguish those who truly need a diagnosis from those who don't. At the extremes of severe illness and complete health, the distinction is indeed obvious. But the boundary between mental disorder and normality is so fuzzy that whenever we quickly expand the use of psychiatric labels to identify some few people who do need help, we misidentify many others who don't.

Human nature is stable and resilient. There has been no real epidemic of mental illness, just a much looser definition of sickness, making it harder for people to be considered well. The people remain the same; the diagnostic labels have changed and are too elastic. Problems that used to be an expected and tolerated part of life are now diagnosed and treated as mental disorder. The application, or withholding, of a sickness label in these boundary situations determines how we see ourselves as individuals and as a society. If we create an overly broad definition and apply it liberally, we readily recruit an army of new "patients," many of whom will have been much better left to their own devices. We are not a sicker society in any real sense—even if we see ourselves that way.

Societal stress is not causing more real mental illness, but there are other societal trends that do promote the sense that we are getting sicker. Our world is homogenizing—we have increasingly less tolerance for individual difference or eccentricity and instead tend to medicalize it into illness. The youngest boy in the class isn't the most active because he is just a young boy—instead he must have ADHD and should be put on a pill.[11] And our society is becoming increasingly perfectionistic. Falling short of complete happiness or failing to have a worry-free life is too often translated into mental illness. Our goals are set too high and our expectations are unrealistic—especially when it comes to our kids.

[handwritten annotation: To some extent. What about those who just realize their sadness is unjustifiable? Sick & tired of being sick & tired. What about increased awareness in society? I mean something in us has changed. Is it strictly behavioral?]

New Fads Promote Diagnostic Inflation

Fashions in psychiatric diagnosis have recently become almost as fickle as the popularity of rock stars, trendy restaurants, and travel destinations. Because there are no biological tests or clear definitions that distinguish normal from mental disorder, everything in psychiatric diagnosis depends on very easily influenced subjective judgments. Whenever rates of a mental disorder jump explosively, the safe bet is always on fad. Assume that many, if not most, of the newly identified "patients" are really "normal enough." They have been mislabeled and will likely be overtreated.

Psychiatric fads start when a powerful authority gives them force and legitimacy. The *DSM* system, and the "experts" who fashioned it, have been the main fashion setters—the driving force in identifying new mental disorders and defining milder forms of those that had been previously described. Unfortunately most experts suffer from an intellectual conflict of interest that biases them toward diagnostic inflation. Focused on their specialized research, they miss the big picture—always worrying so much about not having a diagnosis for a patient who needs one that they ignore the risk of mislabeling someone who doesn't. There is also an emotional element. Experts become true believers who really come to love their pet diagnoses and want to see them grow. While each one presses for only a small expansion, their aggregate pressure blows up the inflationary balloon. In my thirty-five years of herding experts, not once has anyonet ever suggested raising the bar to narrow the scope of his pet area.[12]

The media and the Internet feed on and feed fads. In the wired modern world, false epidemics can be spread like wildfire fueled by the

24/7 coverage. Some of the spotlight is extremely valuable—leading to better public understanding and acceptance of mental disorder, but many stories breathlessly hype diagnostic inflation. "Autism is one in eighty!!!" "The test and cure for Alzheimer's are just around the corner!!!!" "Does your child have ADHD?? "Bipolar is underdiagnosed says Harvard doctor!!!!" And the Internet provides wonderful support, social interaction, information, and destigmatization for people with psychiatric symptoms—but also undercuts normality, as essentially healthy people incorrectly self-identify themselves as sick in order to gain the comforts that come with admittance to the group. Celebrities also play their part as exemplars of diagnoses and endorsers of treatments.

Of course, the biggest promoter of recent fads has been drug company marketing. But that is a sad story in itself that we will get to soon.

DSM Becomes Too Important for Its Own Good

Human nature being what it is, the prevalence of any psychiatric diagnosis will rise artificially whenever it is a gatekeeper to something valuable. In a simpler world, psychiatric diagnosis was once based only on perceived clinical need. But now that it has gained powerful (and unwelcome) influence on many administrative and financial decisions, these decisions have also reciprocally obtained a powerful influence on the rates of diagnosis. Diagnostic inflation is promoted whenever a physician provides an "up-diagnosis" to help a patient gain access to something valuable—like disability benefits or school services. If autism, ADHD, or pediatric bipolar disorder is a prerequisite to being admitted to a small class with lots of individual attention, equivocal cases get shoehorned into these categories, and soon an epidemic is born.

In like fashion, "mental disorder" increases whenever there is high unemployment. Some of the people laid off will get a new diagnosis because they have developed symptoms, others because it will make them eligible for disability. Because veterans' benefits require a diagnosis of PTSD, PTSD gets overdiagnosed. There is a paradox—trying to help by providing a diagnosis may wind up hurting. Many returning vets from Iraq and Afghanistan are having trouble landing jobs because of the stigma associated with their diagnosis of PTSD. And overdiagnosis distorts allocations across the system, reducing resources and benefits for those who most need them.

The most senseless driver of diagnostic inflation is the way medical insurance works in the United States. To get paid, the doctor must make an approved diagnosis. This is intended to prevent frivolous visits. But the unintended effect is just the opposite of prudent cost control. A premature rush to a reimbursable psychiatric diagnosis often results in unnecessary, potentially harmful, and often costly treatment for problems that would have disappeared on their own. It would be a lot cheaper and better for insurance to reimburse the doctor for watchful waiting and counseling, rewarding him for not jumping to diagnostic conclusions that are very costly in the long run. This perfectly sensible solution is the policy in the rest of the world.

Epidemiology Miscounts

Every so often, the newspaper will report that rates of psychiatric disorder are climbing, sometimes dramatically. The best current examples are autism and attention deficit disorder. Don't believe the numbers. The "rates" have been generated by psychiatric epidemiologists, using a method that is inherently flawed and systematically biased in the direction of overreporting.

How can an entire field of scientific endeavor have gone so far astray? It comes down to simple dollar-and-cents considerations. Epidemiological studies have to sample huge numbers of people in the general population, usually using telephone interviews. It would be too expensive to employ clinicians in so extensive an endeavor—so the studies rely on the cheap labor provided by lay interviewers who have no clinical experience and no discretion in judging whether symptoms are clinically meaningful. They make their diagnoses of psychiatric disorders based on symptom counts alone with no consideration of whether the symptoms are severe or enduring enough to really warrant diagnosis or treatment.

This results in rates that are always greatly inflated. Psychiatric symptoms in mild form are widely distributed in the general population—from time to time, almost everyone will have some sadness or anxiety, and others may have difficulty concentrating or be a bit eccentric. But isolated or mild symptoms alone do not define psychiatric disorder—they must cohere over time in a specified way and also cause significant distress or impairment. Epidemiologic studies routinely ignore these crucial requirements. They mistakenly diagnose as psychiatric disorder symptoms that are mild, transient, and lacking in clinical significance.[13]

Results generated in this rough-and-ready way are no more than an upper limit on the prevalence of any given mental disorder. They should never be taken at face value as a true reflection of the real extent of illness in the community. Unfortunately, the exaggerated rates are always reported without proper caveat and are accepted as if they are an accurate reflection of the real prevalence of psychiatric disorder. Disraeli exaggerated only a tad when he said: "There are three kinds of lies: lies, damned lies, and statistics."

The epidemiologists are good bean counters, but they are not clinicians and probably don't know any better. Pharma is less innocent—the results are used to promote the misleading notion that psychiatric disorder is everywhere. The National Institute of Mental Health also likes high rates because they support budget requests to Congress—if mental disorder is everywhere, we should be spending a lot more to research its causes.[14]

Easy-to-Use Drugs Make Excessive Drug Use Far Too Easy

Before the 1950s, the psychotropic drug business was small, and the available drugs were terrible. The opiates and the barbiturates were popular with patients but were nonspecific in their effects and caused big-time problems with addiction and overdose. Bromides, paraldehyde, chloral hydrate, and Miltown were all pretty useless and had hard-to-take side effects.

By the time I began prescribing psychiatric drugs in the 1960s, these old medicines had been mostly superseded by the newly discovered and specific wonder drugs in psychiatry—Thorazine for psychosis, lithium for mania, and Elavil and Nardil for depression. But giving these medicines to patients was still a relatively new thing and a big deal. I trained on the first unit in the United States to use lithium, and we were frankly scared to death of it—an overdose could kill patients or destroy their kidneys, and we were not yet completely sure what were the most effective doses and the safest blood levels. It turned out that the Thorazine doses we were using were way too high and transformed our agitated patients into drugged zombies. The antidepressants available at the time were all extremely risky for use with suicidal outpatients—just a week's worth of pills could be lethal. And they made life miserable for many of the patients taking them—mouth forever parched, bowel movements few and far between, and fainting on standing up a frequent risk. Because the medicines could cause arrhythmias, a fancy cardiac workup had to precede their initiation. Nardil required extremely strict dietary precautions because it interacted dangerously with many foods and with red wine—a little blue cheese, fava beans, or Chianti could be deadly. All of the first psychotropic drugs were so risky and unpleasant to take that only the sickest patients received them, and only well-trained psychiatrists felt comfortable prescribing them.

The next new wave of "wonder" drugs came in the 1970s. The benzodiazepines, Librium and Valium, changed everything and set a new tone—from now on Pharma's emphasis would be on developing and marketing medications that produced less intrusive side effects and were less likely to cause death from overdose. This allowed the focus of care to shift away from the very small cohort of really sick patients to the wider world of the worried well. Before long a large percentage of the U.S. population was taking easy-to-take psychiatric medicine. And because treating patients with "benzos" required no great expertise, primary care physicians took over most of the prescribing. These drugs soon were so wildly successful they became part of the American way of life, and the drug companies realized that psychiatric medicines would become their gold mine. Of course, it turned out that Librium and Valium (and even more, their dreadful younger sib Xanax, introduced in the 1980s) were really quite addicting and not so benign in overdose, particularly when mixed with alcohol or other drugs that depress respiration. They were a great boon to the drug companies, but not to the patients.

Next came the inexorable march of the SSRI antidepressants in the late 1980s and early 1990s—a classic marketing success story. Prozac became a knockout best seller, even spawning a best-selling book by a psychiatrist touting its value not only as an antidepressant but also as a cosmetic drug that could make you better than well.[15] Every year or two thereafter, a new SSRI would appear—Zoloft, Paxil, Celexa—and each would also in turn become a runaway best seller. The marketing of these easy-to-use drugs was closely tied to the marketing of what were (according to the drug companies) easy-to-make psychiatric diagnoses. Soon the SSRIs were also prescribed for panic disorder, generalized anxiety, social phobia, OCD, PTSD, eating disorders, premature ejaculation, and compulsive gambling, and as a general pick-me-up. Sure, there were side effects—some frequent (like reduced sexuality); some rare but dangerous (like agitation, suicidality, and violence). But SSRIs fit so neatly into everyday life that 20 percent of women now take them. Diagnostic inflation will always be an inevitable consequence of an aggressively marketed, easy-to-take pill.

The newer generation of atypical antipsychotics (Risperdal, Zyprexa, Seroquel), introduced in the mid-1990s, are an even more astounding and frightening marketing triumph. Initially they seemed a big step forward—not in efficacy, but in having a much more favorable side effect profile. A patient on traditional antipsychotics had an absolutely characteristic look, easily spotted from far down the hallway—the fixed stare, rigid posture, tremors, abnormal movements, and drooling were dead giveaways. Switched to an atypical, the patient looked and often felt much more normal. Soon these much easier to give and easier to take drugs were climbing to the top of the charts, beating all sales records. This couldn't have been accomplished within the confines of the narrow schizophrenia market. First, the drug companies had to get an indication for bipolar disorder and then they had to advertise a conception of bipolar disorder so broad as to be unrecognizable. Antipsychotics were soon being prescribed promiscuously, even by primary care physicians, to patients with garden-variety anxiety, sleeplessness, and irritability. The paradox is that dangerous drugs capable of causing massive obesity, diabetes, heart disease, and a shortened life span now account for $18 billion a year in sales. Primary care physicians are prescribing potentially dangerous medications, outside their competence, for people who should not be taking them. Proof again that drugs that are too easy to give and too easy to take will be taken far too often, especially when the lots of money is behind them. In retrospect, the unpleasant side effect profiles of early psychiatric drugs had the value of preventing their overuse and of keeping diagnostic inflation in check.

Disease Mongering by Big Pharma

Big Pharma is really big and incredibly successful. Worldwide sales exceed $700 billion each year—half in North America and one fourth in Europe.[16] And the profit margin, at a whopping 17 percent, is among the highest of any industry.[17] Why so big and why so successful? The companies justify their high prices and enormous returns by touting their research efforts to advance medical science and improve patient care. This is mostly fluff. Pharma spends twice as much money ($60 billion) on promotion as on research, and too often they fund the wrong kind of clinical research, done in the wrong way, and with the wrong motives— avoiding lines of inquiry that might actually teach us something important, in favor of surefire "experimercials" that are mostly intended to promote marketing, not discovery.[18]

The surest guarantee of profit is to "me-too" over and over again. Developing a drug that might make a real difference for patients is financially risky. The smarter play for exec bonuses and shareholder dividends is to fiddle slightly with existing compounds—just enough to make them patent-ready lookalikes of compounds already on the gravy train. Companies can double the life of their monopoly patent protection by making the most trivial of changes—turning a right-handed drug to a left-handed one that has identical effects or changing slightly the duration of action. The second surest way to raise revenue and extend patents is to find new market worlds to conquer for an existing drug—by doing research that will get it used by kids or for a diagnosis different from the one originally approved. The market geniuses guide the research effort, not the science types, and the result is predictable—great sales, lousy discovery.

To make matters worse, the research is often performed poorly and presented in an incredibly biased way. The data are proprietary and closely guarded; negative results are routinely buried; tiny, trivial, or chance positive findings are hailed as the second coming; investigators are corrupted; and sometimes scientific papers are ghostwritten by company hacks. Side effects and complications are measured perfunctorily and barely reported. There is never a fair risk/benefit/cost calculus—the benefits are exaggerated, the risks minimized, the costs ignored. Drug pricing has no relation to real cost or value and instead reflects Pharma's monopoly position in the market and its dominance over politicians. At its worst, Pharma research is a deceptive shell game meant to seduce and mislead, rather than enlighten doctors and the public. The claim that drugs are so expensive because they require so much research is pure smoke screen.

A quick review of the last sixty years shows that the drug companies do not have an enviable research record in psychiatry. The most exciting period of discovery in psychopharmacology occurred in the 1950s—and drug company research had absolutely nothing to do with it. The first antipsychotics, first antidepressants, and first mood-stabilizing drugs were all found by pure lone ranger serendipity, a tribute both to the observational skills of their discoverers and to the home-run effectiveness of the drugs. An alert French surgeon noticed that a drug called Thorazine, used preoperatively to prevent nausea, also happened to calm down his patients and made them indifferent to the stress of the procedure. He passed this nugget on to his psychiatrist brother-in-law, and before long the first specific antipsychotic was born. MAO inhibitors that were used to treat tuberculosis were noted to also cheer up the patients, and we had our first antidepressants. And lithium had an unexpected calming effect on laboratory animals that led to its use in mania. None of these breakthroughs was expensive or industrial —all were the product of a good set of eyes and a prepared brain. Like penicillin, the first drug in each class worked so well you didn't really need a double-blind study with hundreds of patients to know that you were on to something big. None of the subsequent sixty years of drug company research has ever once come up with a new product that exceeded the efficacy of the early drugs that were discovered in this way by accident.[19]

Unfortunately, all the low-hanging fruit was picked at the beginning of drug development and the pickings since have been slim and mostly cosmetic. Although late to the starting gate, Pharma quickly caught on to the commercial potential of psychotropic drugs. Many new products were developed and brought to market in the 1960s. The tricyclic antidepressants were an extremely valuable addition to clinical care but had severe limitations as moneymakers because of their troubling side effects and potential for lethal overdose. The real blockbuster breakthrough to the big bucks came when Valium and Librium became household staples. It is an open question whether they contributed more harm or good to patients—they calmed people down but often addicted them and caused all sorts of withdrawal problems. But Pharma had learned a great lesson from them—the real money was in the "user-friendly" medicines that would appeal to a mass consumer market. The SSRIs introduced in the 1980s were the perfect vehicle—no more effective than their predecessors, but much more easily tolerated and safe in overdose. Similarly, the newer antipsychotics were no more effective than their predecessors and carried much worse long-term risks, but were easier to take. This bears repetition—never once has Pharma created a product that exceeded the effectiveness of the drugs available sixty years ago. It has hit many marketing home runs, but usually strikes out when it comes to research. Not an enviable research record after all this time and all this ballyhoo.

Pharma's skills lay elsewhere—it is really ingenious and remarkably effective when it comes to marketing and lobbying. Sixty billion dollars a year will go a long way to sell products and buy politicians. In recent decades, the drug companies have efficiently hijacked the medical enterprise by exerting undue influence on the decisions made by doctors, patients, scientists, journals, professional associations, consumer advocacy groups, pharmacists, insurance companies, politicians, bureaucrats, and administrators. And the best way to sell psychotropic pills is to sell psychiatric ills. Drug companies have many methods of doing this: TV and print media adverts; co-opting most physicians' continuing medical education (often provided at the most expensive restaurants and the nicest resorts; doctors in training and medical students come cheaper—a pizza will do); bankrolling professional associations, journals, and consumer advocacy groups; invading the Internet and social networking sites; recruiting celebrity endorsements. And at one per seven doctors, the drug company sales force (consisting of the most beautiful people this side of Hollywood) has sometimes outnumbered the patients in the waiting room.

Only a very few people have severe mental illness, many more have mild mental illness, but the real mother lode of market share is the worried well. Pharma wants to strip-mine that mother lode and has achieved fantastic revenues by promoting the idea that many of life's expectable problems are mental disorders due to a "chemical imbalance" that can be solved with pill popping. The most creative advertising brains and the most extensive market research help push product into places it had never been before. The pitch to customers is that life is perfectible, if only they will take the simple brain-toning steps to perfect it. The subliminal promise is that beyond curing illness, pills can also help achieve a better way of life through chemistry. If you go to the dentist to correct your less-than-perfect teeth, why not go to the doctor to correct your less-than-perfect brains? No one ever need settle for less than happiness and success. Selling new lifestyles works well for selling cars and beers and perfumes and designer clothing—so why not for selling pills? The message is illustrated with compelling graphic images: the rain stops and the sun shines through when you take an antidepressant; the sad sack becomes the confident leader; the couch potato a well-muscled runner. For kids, the cute little frowning rock becomes the cute little smiling rock. The ads always enjoin us to "Ask your doctor." Of course, the companies have already wired the doctor with a similar message and have provided him with handy free samples to speed you out of the office immediately after you have popped the crucial question.[20]

Many doctors are witting or unwitting agents in the pervasive drug company marketing campaign to sell new diagnoses. "Education" and "research" can become sheep's clothing covering what is really a wolfish marketing pitch. A large stable of psychiatry's "thought leaders" are recruited to help drumbeat the wondrous benefits that accrue from drugs and to downplay the harms. Things are becoming better now, but for a time Pharma used thought leaders to exert dominance over psychiatry's educational and research programs. The dozens of industry-sponsored symposia at the annual meeting of the American Psychiatric Association offered the best speakers and the only food and attracted the biggest audiences. Most of weekly grand rounds held at hospitals and medical schools throughout the country were funded by Pharma and led by big-name faculty conveniently supplied by its "speakers' bureaus."

I know about the "thought leader" issue firsthand because I used to be one. My participation with the pharmaceutical industry goes back thirty years and has taken a variety of forms. In the 1980s, I was vice-chair of the APA program committee responsible for organizing its annual meetings. I went along with a group decision to accept drug-company-sponsored symposia—made on the grounds that the topics and speakers offered would be of interest to the membership—not anticipating that before long these would become so popular as to completely overshadow the rest of the meetings and so biased as to be more commercial than disinterested science. For fifteen years I was director of an outpatient clinic at Cornell that occasionally performed drug-company-sponsored research studies. Many of the thousand or more talks I have given over the years were financed directly or indirectly by drug company money. I developed a series of expert consensus guidelines that were industry funded. And as chair of psychiatry at Duke University I presided over a department that had extensive industry sponsorship for a number of its research and educational programs. In none of these activities did I ever once say or publish anything I did not believe to be completely accurate, and I often said and published things that made drug company representatives wince with pain. I always recognized the risk that hidden strings could be attached and don't think I was ever restrained by them to present things in a biased way. But in retrospect, it was unseemly to have participated in so many activities that could be construed as indirect drug marketing. And I saw the slippery slope facing those who had a deeper involvement and fewer scruples.

If everyone has the ill, then all must take the pill.[21] Already huge, the market in psychotropic drugs is constantly growing. When the adult market seemed saturated, the drug companies expanded their customer demographics by pushing product onto children—it is not by accident that all the recent epidemics of psychiatric disorder have occurred in kids. And children are particularly choice customers—bring them on board early, and you may have them for life. At the other end of the life cycle, companies targeted the elderly, selling antipsychotics like hotcakes in nursing homes. Pharma has not been constrained by the fact that children and the elderly are the two most difficult demographic groups to diagnose accurately or that they are the most vulnerable to harmful drug side effects or that excessive use of antipsychotics in nursing homes results in increased mortality. And, even more troubling, it is the very most vulnerable of kids who get the most medicine—those who are economically disadvantaged or in foster care.[22]

Seven percent of Americans are now addicted to a legal psychotropic drug.[23] Prescription drug abuse has become a bigger problem than illicit drug abuse. If there is a conceivable way to sell a new diagnosis so that people will incorrectly believe they have it, drug companies will have figured it out and will do it successfully—if sometimes illegally. Big Pharma seems to feel above the law. Almost all of the companies have absorbed huge fines and even criminal penalties as punishment for their illegal sales practices.[24] Drugs are approved by the Food and Drug Administration only for the treatment of those mental disorders for which studies indicate there is sufficient efficacy and safety. Although doctors are given the discretion to prescribe a medicine "off-label" for other uses, it is strictly illegal for drug companies to encourage them to do so. The drug company "Hall of Shame" (see below) shows how flagrantly Pharma flouts the law. A seemingly hefty fine of $1.3 billion may be no more than affordable chump change and the cost of doing business, considering the enormous revenues that can be earned through shady marketing. Only much bigger fines and tighter regulations can tame this beast. And doctors should be cautioned that

DRUG COMPANY HALL OF SHAME

PREPARED BY MELISSA RAVEN PhD

DATE	COMPANY	FINES/SETTLEMENTS	DRUG(S)	CULPABLE ACTS
August 2012	Johnson & Johnson	$181 million civil	Risperdal	Off-label promotion[25]
July 2012	GlaxoSmith-Kline	$3 billion: $1 billion criminal, $2 billion civil	Paxil, Wellbutrin, Avandia	Off-label promotion; failure to report safety data (Avandia)[26]
May 2012	Abbott	$1.5 billion: $700 million criminal, $800 million civil	Depakote	Off-label promotion[27]
April 2012	Johnson & Johnson	$1.1 billion criminal	Risperdal	Off-label promotion to children and elderly; fraudulent marketing tactics[28]
January 2012	Johnson & Johnson	$158 million	Risperdal	Off-label promotion, misrepresentation of safety[29]
September 2010	Novartis	$422.5 million: $185 million criminal, $237.5 million civil	Trileptal	Off-label promotion, for bipolar disorder, neuropathic pain[30]
September 2010	Forest	$313 million: $164 million criminal, $149 million civil	Lexapro, Celexa, Levothroid	Off-label promotion, for children and adolescents; false claims; distribution of unapproved drug (Levothroid)[31]
April 2010	AstraZeneca	$520 million civil	Seroquel	Off-label promotion, targeting geriatricians, PCPs, pediatricians[32]
September 2009	Pfizer	$1.3 billion criminal, $1 billion civil	Geodon, Lyrica, Bextra, Zyvox	Off-label marketing[33]
January 2009	Eli Lilly	$1.415 billion: $515 billion criminal, $800 million civil	Zyprexa	Off-label promotion, for dementia, agitation, aggression, hostility, depression, and generalized sleep disorder[34]
September 2007	Bristol-Myers Squibb	$515 million civil	Abilify, Serzone, among others	Illegal marketing and pricing; off-label promotion[35]
July 2007	Purdue	Nearly $635 million civil fines, penalties, and restitution payments, $500,000 criminal	OxyContin	Fraudulent misbranding, causing false claims to be filed[36]
2004	Warner-Lambert (Pfizer)	$430 million: $240 million criminal, $190 million civil	Neurontin	Off-label promotion, for bipolar disorder, pain, migraine, alcohol withdrawal[37]

off-label prescribing is out of control, is often harmful, and sometimes constitutes a form of malpractice.

Placebo Response Sells Pills

The word *placebo* comes from the Latin meaning "I please." And do placebos ever please. The "placebo effect" refers to people getting better because of positive expectations independent of any specific healing effect of the treatment. The placebo effect is very effective— people routinely get great results from treatments that have nothing whatever to do with their illness. It is probably fair to say that placebo is the greatest broad-spectrum wonder drug ever invented—cheap, effective for almost all but the most severe of man's ills, and with very few side effects.

But the placebo effect also causes a very serious problem—it keeps people taking expensive, and sometimes harmful, pills they don't need for conditions they don't have. The history of medicine is littered with dreadful treatments that were often much more dangerous than the diseases they were meant to cure. Magical thinking has allowed doctors to inflict (and patients to accept) great harm while claiming illusory benefits—the doctor's orders dutifully followed even when completely ineffective or quite hurtful. Long-suffering patients have been given emetics to help them vomit up their sickness; purgatives to help them defecate it; leeches to suck it out; and skull holes to release it. They were dunked to the point of almost drowning; subjected to high fevers; wrapped in cold packs; and spun in special chairs or from ropes hanging from the ceiling. All sorts of substances we now fear greatly as highly toxic poisons were once treasured as healing nostrums. The placebo effect is the only way to explain this rogue's gallery of what now seem obviously silly, even sinister treatments that have caused millennia of needless additional suffering to people who were already sick enough to begin with. The placebo effect is a kind of medical magic that gives doctors an undeserved authority and accounts for their frequent belief in really bad treatments.

The wonders of placebo response arise from a number of different causes—sometimes independent, sometimes interacting. Most important perhaps is "tincture of time." Time may not always be the best healer and it certainly doesn't heal all wounds, but it always has been and still is the most efficient and safest way to deal with many of life's physical and psychological problems. Time heals so well because many of our ills are short-term, situational, and self-limited—our bodies and our minds are programmed to be resilient without any active effort on our part.

Next comes the enormous power of hope and expectation. People get better if they believe in a treatment and have full confidence that it will help them get better—however irrelevant or even dangerous it may be. Life has always been painful and perilous. The power of positive thinking is part of our psychology because it has conferred such a strong selective advantage on those fortunate enough to have it. Perhaps the swift had the early edge in the evolutionary race, but it was the enduring who made it to the finish line—and survived to become our ancestors. Being able to overcome the discouragements and disadvantages of illness by responding well to fake medicine was a sure path to evolutionary success.

Brain imaging proves that the placebo effect has strong biological as well as psychological roots. My favorite example comes from wine tasting, not medicine. It has long been known that people routinely rate a wine as much better if they are told it costs ninety dollars a bottle, rather than ten dollars. This proves how suggestible we are. But brain imaging tells us something even more fascinating and fundamental about human nature. Your brain's pleasure centers actually light up more when you think you are drinking the costlier wine, even if you're not. Expectation isn't all of experience, but it certainly does shape a goodly portion of it. Similarly, placebo pain pills dampen the brain's response to painful stimuli; placebo antidepressants mimic the brain effects of real antidepressants; placebo Parkinson's pills stimulate the brain's dopamine system; placebo diabetes pills affect blood sugar; placebo caffeine and Ritalin have a stimulating impact on brain centers; and placebos profoundly affect the immune system. Placebo response is an important part of our reaction to everything. And it is very deeply built into the way our brains work—animals are also terrific placebo responders.

The social factor is also important—being a placebo responder helps maintain key relationships and supports precious communal rituals. We are highly social animals who function well only as part of a group and who threaten the group's welfare when we are not functioning well. The medicine man and his patients have always shared the need to believe in the healing power of the currently fashionable theories, rituals, chants, incantations, diagnostic and testing procedures, and medicines. Even if it had no specific value, a healing ritual offers the great promise of ridding the individual of his illness and the group of the sicknesses in its individuals. Responding well to placebo is essential to remaining a valued member of the group—which made it less likely you would be left behind as too sick when everyone broke camp. And being able to enlist the confidence and hope of the sick patient has always been and still is the most essential skill in a great shaman or a great modern doctor. The technical skills of medicine are becoming increasingly routine and may soon be done better by computer programs—but the shamanic skills of medicine will always be important to patients and to society.

Modern drug companies have made big bucks capitalizing on the power and ubiquity of the placebo response. The best way to get great results with a pill is to treat people who don't really need it—the highest placebo response rates occur in those who would get better naturally and on their own.[38,39] The really brilliant marketing trick was to persuade doctors to treat patients who weren't really sick, while at the same time convincing normal people that they were really sick. Expanding market share to include the worried well not only greatly enhanced the customer pool, but it also ensured the most satisfied of customers. Placebo responders often become long-term loyalists to medication use even when the medication is perfectly useless, both because they have no way of knowing it played no role in their getting better and because they are often untroubled by side effects—a cunning combination that creates the dream customer base for drug companies and their shareholders.

In surveys, most doctors admit to sometimes using relatively inoffensive pills as placebos—a way of giving the patient something tangible on the way out the door.[40] If the prescribing of placebos was ever accepted as ethical practice, they would undoubtedly rise to the very top of the sales charts. To paraphrase Voltaire, the art of medicine sometimes consists in amusing the patient while nature cures the disease.

In veiled form, placebos are already the great, if unrecognized, success story of drug company marketing. A good deal of medication use in psychiatry (and in medicine) is based on the tried-and-true leveraging of the placebo effect. There are only two differences between now and shaman times or medieval alchemy. First, the marketing of what are essentially expensive placebo products has become well-oiled, massively financed, worldwide, and devastatingly effective. Second, you now need to have a *DSM* diagnosis to get a prescription for an expensive pill that often has no more usefulness than would a placebo—a great boost to diagnostic inflation. And the crowning irony is that, like wine tasting, it may be that the higher the price, the more effective the otherwise useless pill. How great for the drug companies.

Two brilliant marketing successes illustrate the financial as well as healing, power of placebo. Almost three fourths of the 11 percent of the U.S. population now taking antidepressant drugs have no current symptoms of depression.[41] Some of these people would soon get quite sick again were they to stop the pills—they need them as prophylactic protection against the return of a chronic or recurring depression. But many loyal customers are unwitting placebo responders who got well spontaneously (but don't know it) and are afraid to rock the boat. A significant portion of the $12 billion spent each year on antidepressants in the United States rewards the drug companies for promoting the overly widespread use of what to many patients are no more than highly advertised, oversold, and very expensive placebos prescribed for a fake diagnosis.

And here's another case in point—the strange success story of Buspar, how it became one of the surprise best-selling drugs of all time despite having little or no efficacy. When Buspar first came on the market, I told its drug company executive that it surely would be a huge flop because it didn't work. He said nothing but smiled knowingly, probably because he understood something that was beyond my naive comprehension. The seeming great disadvantage of having little (if any) efficacy against anxiety was more than counterbalanced by Buspar's also having almost no side effects. Being the perfect, easy-to-use, and expensive placebo was just the right prescription for bringing in huge profits.

Let's do an interesting thought experiment. Suppose we could eliminate the magic of placebo response, or at least reduce through education its impact on patient behavior. The immediate effects would be both bad and good—dramatically reduced perceived efficacy of many medicines, but also dramatically reduced unnecessary diagnosis and treatment. Of course, this thought experiment will never become real—magical thinking is too much a necessary and useful part of human nature. But it would be nice if people could be more skeptical of drug company claims that the worries and miseries of everyday life are just a "chemical imbalance" that can be cured with a pill.

Im confused ...

How Primary Care Took Over Much of Psychiatry

Primary care physicians (PCPs) now do most of the prescribing of psychiatric drugs: 90 percent of antianxiety drugs; 80 percent of antidepressants; 65 percent of stimulants; and 50 percent of antipsychotics.[42]

Pharma did the math—there are only forty thousand psychiatrists in the United States but about ten times as many PCPs. Why not recruit PCPs to write prescriptions for psychiatric drugs? The message to them was loud, clear, and heavily promoted—psychiatric disorders are often missed and easy to treat with a magic pill. This was clinical nonsense but marketing gold. The message went down easily because the new pills went down easily—with relatively few immediately troubling side effects for patients and uncomplicated directions for use by doctors. Who needs a psychiatrist when the medicine is so safe and easy to use? Insurance companies pitched in by preferring PCPs over psychiatrists because they were cheaper (at least in the short run), especially once they were squeezed by diminishing reimbursements into doing seven-minute visits.

Anywhere between 25 to 50 percent of patients seen in primary care present with at least some emotional distress as part of the reason for coming to the doctor.[43] Most of the patients treated by PCPs have mild disorders—precisely the ones most likely to have a placebo response. Once recovered, the patient will usually misattribute his improvement to a medicine that did nothing and feel compelled to stay on it unnecessarily and for prolonged periods. This represents the perfect market opportunity—an army of patients primed by advertising to ask the doctor for a pill. And the doctor primed to respond promptly, since most of his education in psychiatry had come from the helpful drug company salesperson—who also happened to have a handy supply of free samples. Harried PCPs are underpaid and overworked, and have minimal training in psychiatry. Convenience sometimes trumps good care, and the quickest way for them to speed the patient out of the office is to reach for prescription pad or free sample. Psychiatric medications can do a lot of good when properly prescribed, but a lot of harm when handed out so casually and after such incomplete diagnostic evaluations.

The inevitable result has been diagnostic inflation and massively excessive medication use. It makes absolutely no sense to do most of our psychiatric diagnosis and treatment in primary care settings. Accurate diagnosis requires expertise and simply can't be done properly in the seven minutes most PCPs now get to spend with patients—especially when the patients have been primed by false advertising to demand the wrong thing. Overprescription of psychotropic medication by PCPs has become a serious threat to public health, but has pushed Pharma revenue through the roof. There is almost never a justification for the use of antipsychotic and antianxiety medication in primary care, but it is done all the time.

The fault lays mostly with the system, not the doctor. Ideally primary care should be the valued linchpin central to all medical treatment; instead, our skewed specialist-happy care delivery has left it devalued and terribly underfunded. PCPs man the crucial entry point to the healing world and are forced to deal with the widest array of medical, surgical, and psychiatric problems—a very tall order indeed. Often the PCP is the caregiver with best overall and longest term familiarity with the patient and the one to whom the patient goes for the aches and pains of his life as well as his body. He is the health provider of first, and perhaps last, resort, as often the patient can't afford specialty care or it may be unavailable.[44] Some PCPs handle their role as "psychiatrists" beautifully, but many are dangerous amateurs who do more harm than good—especially when they arettt pressured by the misleading drug company marketing and are forced to shoot from the hip by insurance industry time constraints.

Bad Consequences of Diagnostic Inflation

Where Have All the Normals Gone?

In the early 1980s, about a third of Americans qualified for a lifetime diagnosis of mental disorder.[45] Now about half do.[46] And Europe is catching up fast at well over 40 percent.[47] Some people think these are underestimates—more carefully done prospective studies actually double the lifetime prevalence. If you believe the results, our population is almost totally saturated with mental disorders. One study found that by age thirty-two, 50 percent of the general population had already qualified for an anxiety disorder; more than 40 percent for mood disorder; and more than 30 percent for substance dependence.[48] And another study moved even closer to the proposition of almost ubiquitous sickness—by the tender age of twenty-one, more than 80 percent of young adults had already met criteria for a mental disorder.[49] The trumpeting of inflated rates has fueled drug company claims that we are underdiagnosed and undertreated—keeping the vicious cycle spinning.

Evidence of diagnostic inflation is everywhere. There have been four explosive epidemics of mental disorder in the past fifteen years. Childhood bipolar disorder increased by a miraculous fortyfold[50]; autism by a whopping twentyfold[51]; attention deficit/hyperactivity has tripled[52]; and adult bipolar disorder doubled.[53] Whenever rates skyrocket, some portion of the rise represents previously missed true cases—people who really need the diagnosis and the treatment that follows from it. But more accurate diagnosis can't explain why so many people, especially kids, suddenly seem to be getting so sick.

The Glut of Drugs

Psychotropic drugs are now among the very top best sellers for the drug companies. Their stock prices would be cut by more than half were it not for the antipsychotics, antidepressants, stimulants, anti-anxiety agents, sleeping pills, and pain meds Each year, 300 million prescriptions are written for psychiatric drugs in the United States alone.[54] At the very top of the Pharma hit parade are the antipsychotics at a resounding $18 billion a year. Antidepressants produce a hardy $12 billion a year, despite the fact that many are now off patent and sold in cheaper generic versions. Fifteen years ago, stimulants were a rounding error in drug company sales at a measly $50 million a year. Now with direct-to-consumer advertising and heavy marketing to doctors, sales have been juiced up to a hefty $8 billion a year.[55] And because primary care doctors love to prescribe them, antianxiety agents are eighth in sales among drug classes—even though they probably do much more harm than good.

The biggest puzzle is the huge success of antipsychotic drugs. Despite their dangerous side effects and narrow indications, they are being given out like candy. Antipsychotics have proven usefulness only in treating the disabling symptoms of schizophrenia and bipolar disorder, but this has not stopped drug company seduction promoting their general use for anyone having trouble sleeping, or run-of-the-mill anxiety, or depression, or irritability, or eccentricity, or the temper tantrums of youth, or the crankiness of old age. More than 3 million Americans are already on board, with a (shareholder satisfying) growth rate of 20 percent a year. The number of prescriptions for antipsychotics has doubled in ten years, up to 54 million and counting. Off-label use has also doubled—undeterred by the big fines that don't seem so big when you consider the ill-gotten gains they enable. How could this happen? Big bucks. An advertising budget of $2.4 billion per year spent on Abilify and Seroquel has catapulted these two very so-so and not-so-safe drugs to fifth and sixth place as revenue producers among all of the many medicines sold in America. The full court press on primary care doctors has them inappropriately prescribing an antipsychotic for 20 percent of all their anxiety disorder patients.[56, 57, 58] This massive misuse of antipsychotics is crazy and shameful—a triumph of marketing might over common sense and good medical practice.

There is no way of knowing what should be the optimal level of prescription drug use in our society. Enthusiasts argue that the high rates of pill taking reflect the advances in psychiatric diagnosis and treatment—providing benefits heretofore unavailable to people previously ignored and in need. To some degree, this is true. But I have no doubt there has been a wild overshoot of false demand promoted by false drug company advertising, gullible doctors, careless prescribing habits, and the wholesale transfer of psychiatric diagnosis and treatment to untrained and harried primary care doctors. We have become a pill-popping society, and very often it is the wrong people who are popping the wrong pills as prescribed by the wrong doctors.

Its undue influence over medical practice is not Big Pharma's fault; it is ours. A drug company does not begin life or maintain itself as a nonprofit or charitable entity chartered with the goal of promoting public health in the most efficient and effective way. Quite the opposite. A drug company is a multinational corporation whose main goals are profit, market share, and survival. In any conflict between shareholder greed and customer need, bet on the shareholder. This is the predatory nature of the beast—it is not the tiger's fault it is a carnivore. But it is our collective fault for allowing the drug companies free rein to prey on our weakness. Government, doctors, patients, the media, advocacy groups—all were largely bought off by drug company money and power. Drugs used well are a powerful tool of psychiatry and a godsend for the patients helped. But too often, drugs are used promiscuously in a way that approximates the quackish practice of medieval alchemists. Thomas Sydenham must have had in mind trigger-happy prescribers when he said: "The arrival of a good clown exercises a more beneficial influence upon the health of a town than twenty asses laden with drugs."

Too Much Polypharmacy

It has become distressingly common for doctors to prescribe multiple psychotropic drugs, often in high and dangerous doses and without any rhyme or reason. It is no surprise that drugs prescribed by doctors now account for more emergency room visits for overdoses than do street drugs and are also increasingly responsible for accidental iatrogenic deaths.[5] The interacting sedating side effects of the combination of narcotic pain medicine and psychotropic drugs can be especially deadly (a particular problem in the military).[60]

There are many tributaries to this surging river of polypharmacy. Sometimes it represents treatment creep—the previous drugs aren't working very well so new ones keep getting added without ever sunsetting the ineffective ones. Sometimes it results from diagnostic creep—exuberance in making multiple diagnoses followed by enthusiasm in prescribing multiple medications. Sometimes the cause is doctor creep—a drug-seeking patient getting all the meds he can from different doctors blind to one another's prescriptions. Then there is Pharma creep—aggressive marketing that encourages promiscuous prescription. And finally, there is the easy availability of diverted prescription drugs, which encourages polypharmacy by self-prescription—people who decide to add their friend's stimulant or Xanax or narcotic pain medicine to their own often already bloated treatment regimen.

Some doctors seem to use the same combination of medications on every patient, regardless of symptom presentation. The prescribed doses are sometimes high enough to cause serious problems on their own and are especially dangerous if the patient pushes the envelope by drinking alcohol, using drugs, or even taking a few extra pills. The wildest prescribers tend to accumulate deaths over the years, usually without inviting much-needed discipline or increased supervision.

All this said, polypharmacy is sometimes rational and even necessary. The combination of antipsychotic and antidepressant works much better than either alone in treating bipolar disorder or psychotic depression. When a patient has had a definite but partial response to one drug, another may be needed to get a full response. And rarely does adding a pill for sleep make sense. But most polypharmacy is unnecessary, unsupported by research, unmonitored, harmful, and even dangerous.

Too Little Psychotherapy

There is no organized psychotherapy industry to mount a concerted competitive push-back against the excessive use of drugs. Psychotherapy is a retail, individualized, preindustrial craft that doesn't lend itself to the wholesale industrial standardization of product and people that has been so lucrative for Pharma. The different psychotherapies and their practitioners are extremely fragmented and lack the financial resources needed to break the drug company monopoly of the airwaves. Talk doesn't pay—psychiatrists who provide psychotherapy along with medication during a forty-five-minute outpatient visit earn 41 percent less than do psychiatrists who provide three fifteen-minute medication management sessions.[61] The percentage of visits to psychiatrists that included psychotherapy dropped from 44 percent in 1996 to 1997, to 29 percent in 2004 to 2005.[62,63]

Psychotherapy also lacks a unified, catchy message to counter the seductively misleading drug company promo "it is all chemical imbalance." But psychotherapy does have a much more important and truthful story to tell—that it performs as well as drugs when compared head-to-head in people with mild to moderately severe problems.[64, 65, 66] Though psychotherapy takes a bit longer to work and costs more upfront, it has more enduring beneficial effects, and that may make it cheaper and better in the long run than long-term medication. Taking a pill is passive. In contrast, psychotherapy puts the patient in charge by instilling new coping skills and attitudes toward life. Japan has caught on to this advantage. Until recently, all of its psychiatric treatment was medication based, but now the government is making a concerted national effort to break the drug monopoly by promoting cognitive therapy as an alternative—because it works well and is cost-effective.

The Power to Label Is the Power to Destroy *stigma*

Merriam-Webster defines the word *stigma* as an identifying mark, a specific diagnostic sign of disease, or a scar or spot on a plant or animal. Some dictionaries even use "the stigma of mental illness" as the best specific example of the disadvantages suffered by those who are marked. Being "normal" and fitting in with the pack are a key to survival. Evolution has wired into human nature an uncharitable wariness and lack of compassion for those who are different and don't satisfy tribal standards.

Having a mental disorder label "marks" someone in ways that can cause much secondary harm.[67] Stigma takes many forms, comes from all directions, is sometimes blatantly overt, but can also be remarkably subtle. It is the cruel comment, the unkind smirk, the extrusion from the group, the lost job opportunity, the rejected marriage proposal, the ineligibility for life insurance, the inability to adopt a child or pilot a plane. But it is also the reduced expectation, the helping hand when none is needed or wanted, the solicitous sympathy that one cannot really be expected to measure up. And the secondary psychological and practical harms of having a mental disorder come only partly from how others see you. A great deal of the trouble comes from a change in how you see yourself—the sense of being damaged goods, feeling not normal or worthy, not a full-fledged member of the group.

It is bad enough that stigma is so often associated with having a mental disorder. But the stigma that comes from being mislabeled with a fake diagnosis is a dead loss with absolutely no redeeming features. Labels can also create self-fulfilling prophecies. If you are told you are sick, you feel and act sick, and others treat you as if you are sick. The sick role can be enormously useful when someone truly is sick and needs respite and care. But the sick role can be extremely destructive when it reduces expectations, truncates ambitions, and results in a loss of personal responsibility.[68]

And when a society allows the overdiagnosis of a significant proportion of its individuals as "sick," it becomes an artificially "sick" society rather than a resolutely resilient one. Our ancestors lived through wars and privations unimaginable to us—without resorting to an overdose of labels and an overuse of pills.

Turning Bad into Mad

Diagnostic inflation is an ever-present danger at the boundary between psychiatry and the law. "I would rather be hung as a man than acquitted as a fool." So screamed Charles Guiteau to the jury during his trial for the assassin of President James Garfield in 1881.[69] He was renouncing the insanity defense offered by his lawyers—preferring instead to be seen as a messenger of God sent to save the United States from an evil administration. Better to be convicted as a criminal than absolved as a mental patient because this would reduce the credibility of his claims. Setting a precedent that continues to this day, many doctors testified on both sides of this landmark case—some seeing Guiteau as crazed, others as a sane, if misguided, criminal.

This debate rages on with no solution. Are political terrorists like the Unabomber or the Norwegian mass murderer Anders Breivik best considered political criminals or mental patients? When assassins strike public figures or innocent bystanders, the media always questions whether they are crazy, never wonders how much they were egged on by venomous political discourse or how they so easily got that semiautomatic. Many (perhaps most) political assassins and mass murderers are on the fuzzy boundary between the merely strange and the legally insane. Depending on your perspective, they can plausibly be seen as either violent political or religious extremists or as delusional psychotics. The adversarial testimony of expert psychiatric witnesses on both sides of this divide invariably cancels out. Ultimately it is a societal, not a medical, choice, whether to consider such individuals mad or bad. Most defendants would, like Guiteau, much prefer to be punished than treated—lest their message be muffled. I would agree with them. Except in the clearest cases to the contrary, diagnostic inflation should be tamed in the courts. Bad should usually trump mad.

opinion —   *... ?*

Paying the Bill for Diagnostic Inflation

No one has calculated the total direct and indirect monetary costs of diagnostic inflation, but it must add up to a vast fortune of wasted resources. First, there is the cost of all the unnecessary and overpriced drugs and the doctors' visits needed to prescribe them. Add to this the downstream costs that arise from the many and expensive complications that arise from excessive drug use. In the short term, this includes the costly emergency room visits and hospitalizations for overdoses. Then there are the long-run massive but hidden costs of treating the medical and psychiatric complications caused by medication use—most especially the secondary obesity, diabetes, and heart disease. And how do we cost the lost years of life for those who die early because of the harmful short-term or long-term impact of unnecessary drugs?

Next we have to add the cost of lost work productivity. Linking psychiatric diagnosis to disability artificially inflates both—those who are mislabeled are more likely to become absentees or to stop working altogether. Holland and Denmark discovered that national sick days and disability skyrocketed when a psychiatric diagnosis or work stress was a readily accepted reason for not working. The disability decision is often an irrevocable moment in a person's life: gaining disability is a wonderful short-term respite from terribly worrying financial pressures, but it may lead to chronic vocational invalidism.

Then there are the costs of other services provided to people mislabeled as mentally ill—the mental health and medical visits, the added school services, training programs, and so on. It seems harsh to begrudge these to anyone, and in the individual case a caring clinician will be tempted to up-diagnose to help his own patient get the benefit. But budgets are usually a zero-sum game—helping this person who has only a marginal need will mean depriving someone else who has a crying-out-loud need.

Finally, we come to the forensic and correctional costs of diagnostic inflation. A single death penalty sentencing hearing can cost $5 million for endless and futile debates on the presence or absence of a highly dubious mental disorder. A year in a psychiatric hospital for someone inappropriately committed under an SVP statute costs more than a year at Harvard. Civil lawsuits based on creative claims of psychiatric damage drag on seemingly forever and eat up treasures in legal bills and fees for expert witnesses. Psychiatry and the law often don't mix well—but they always cost a lot whenever they become entangled.

The enormous waste caused by diagnostic inflation goes unchecked because there are no feedback controls to contain it and no economic incentives to promote careful diagnosis. Waste never enters into the considerations of those who develop the DSMs or those who apply it or to the drug companies who profit from it. Parents understandably want services for their child and consumer advocacy groups understandably want services for their constituents. It always appears that someone else is paying the bill and no one is minding the store to ensure rational and fair allocations. The net result is inevitable: unnecessary demand created by diagnostic inflation results in wasted expenditures, while those in desperate need remain badly underserved.[70]

Diagnostic inflation is a public health and public policy dilemma that urgently needs solving. Costs will be further amplified by the extension of health insurance to some 34 million more Americans under the Affordable Care Act, especially given its requirement that insurance include comprehensive care for mental disorders. These are wonderful policy changes. A greater investment is certainly needed to shore up our badly shortchanged mental health system. But the additional expenditures are unpredictable, likely to be in the many billions each year, and because of diagnostic inflation, the money will be spent where it is likely to do least good.

Curing diagnostic inflation will be an uphill struggle, with steps to be described later. But first we have to understand the large role diagnostic fads have played in the psychiatric past, the grave damage they are doing in the present, and the significant risk that new fads will create mayhem in the immediate future.

PART II

Psychiatric Fads Can Be Bad for Your Health

CHAPTER 4

Fads of the Past

We don't see things as they are. We see things as we are.
TALMUD

FADS IN PSYCHIATRIC diagnosis come and go. All of a sudden everyone seems to have the same problem. Quack theories explain the outbreak; quack treatments presume to provide cure. Then, equally suddenly, the epidemic runs its course and the once ubiquitous diagnosis disappears from circulation.[1]

Fads depend on the combination of a plausible idea and our copycat, follow-the-leader herd instinct. Like stock market fluctuations, they are probably most common during times of instability, uncertainty, and change. The causes can be deep and general to the human condition or quite specific to a given historical development, the publication of a popular book or movie, or a new medical treatment. Some of the misleading ways of understanding psychiatric disorder have lasted for millennia, others only for decades. Demonic possession is so powerful and plausible an explanation for strange feelings, thoughts, and behaviors that it recurs at all times and in all places. Multiple personality disorder is a much less satisfying fad—it pops up only rarely and never lasts very long.

People don't really change much, but labels do. Humanity's symptoms and behaviors may oscillate a bit but probably remain basically stable over time. In contrast, the way we characterize them can fluctuate as wildly as changing fashions in music or hemlines. The symptoms and suffering are real—but sometimes we get trapped by explanations and labels that are just plain wrong and far too convincing.

Being aware of fads of the past will help us be skeptical about whatever has become a "diagnosis du jour" in the present. The best antidote to following foolish current or future fashion is appreciating how harmful previous fashions have been. History never precisely repeats itself because its complex interactions are pregnant with probabilistic permutations. But history does have to rhyme, because the underlying forces shaping it are fairly stable, even if outward appearances are in apparent flux. The more we know the rhymes of the past, the less likely we are to mindlessly repeat them in the future.

Demonic Possession (Circa: Then, Now, and Always)

Demonic possession is the oldest of fads and the newest; it is recorded in the earliest written documents and reported in today's newspaper. Belief in devils may be the fruit of ignorance—but it is too appealing a model ever to disappear from human belief and provides stiff competition to the slender comforts of rational thought, mainstream religion, and psychiatry. It will always be with us in one form or another and every so often explodes into a fad, sometimes with devastating results.[2]

The real beauty of demonic possession is that it not only describes the problems but also provides a compelling explanation of their cause and a ready suggestion for their cure. A demon has possessed the person, taking control of his thoughts, feelings, and behaviors and causing a whole grab bag of symptoms that could be divided into at least a dozen different *DSM* mental disorders. Today's psychiatrist can describe schizophrenia, but can't begin to explain it. The medicine man or priest is in a much more powerful position. He has sure knowledge of what is causing the symptoms and a specific treatment intended to separate the patient from the disease. Exorcising the demon can work well when the exorcist and the patient both believe it will.

The belief in demonic control is universal across cultures and enduring through time because it makes so much sense to most people; it taps into something basic in human psychology and explains a large part of human experience in a simple and plausible way. The battle against demons appeals to the theological mind; cures most of the symptoms that ail us; ministers to the soul; and binds the tribe. Demons are a completely logical, if prescientific, way of understanding the changes caused by psychiatric and medical illness (and also by drugs, dreams, and trance states). It appears silly only to us children of the Enlightenment who believe in biological causes of strange behavior. But there is one unavoidable problem with this otherwise useful diagnostic category—it has provided a wonderful excuse for the persecution, torture, and murder of the mentally ill. The very most inhumane treatment could easily be justified on the spurious grounds that it was part of a holy fight against the devil.

Modern psychiatric diagnosis and demonic possession could be seen as opposite ways of explaining the causality of troubled behavior—disease of the brain versus disease caused by spirits. Most people in the developed world are more comfortable with modern science. But not all. More than a third of Americans believe that demons and angels play an active role in their daily lives. And worried that victims of possession are being misdiagnosed by psychiatrists as schizophrenic, modern-day exorcists have posted detailed Internet diagnostic manuals teaching how to spot the devil in the disease. The Catholic Church is less radical in its belief in demons, recommending exorcism only when the symptoms are specific to sacrilege and after mental illness has been ruled out. Outbreaks of demonic possession occur all the

time in war-torn Africa. The latest epidemic in the United States occurred twenty years ago as part of the hysteria around "satanic ritual
abuse."

Dance Manias: Tarantism and Saint Vitus's Dance (Circa: 1300 to 1700)

Dance manias came in two quite similar forms: tarantism in southern
Italy and Saint Vitus's dance in northern Europe. The symptoms were
some combination of melancholy, visions, headache, fainting, breath-
lessness, twitching, loss of appetite, soreness, swelling, and premoni-
tions of imminent death. In the south these were attributed to the bite
of the tarantula, endemic to the area. Onset was usually during the
height of midsummer, and heat was presumed to enhance the toxic effects. Saint Vitus's dance was a northern European variant with many
of the same symptoms, cured in the same way, but with a more religious cast.

Regardless of cause, the recommended treatment was a freneti-
cally rapid, deliriously dizzying, whirling dance, to be continued to the
point of physical exhaustion and mental rejuvenation. Dancing was
presumed to remove the spiders' poison (in the south) or the demon
from the soul (in the north). Tens, or hundreds, or even thousands
of people would participate jointly in a group epidemic and cure that
would last continuously for hours, days, or even weeks. Alcohol was
used in large quantities and sleep deprivation also played a role. As
is also true today, it was often difficult to separate the side effects of
the treatment from the symptoms of the illness. People would behave
strangely, tear off clothing, scream, squeal, laugh or weep uncontrollably, be openly sexual, and make animal gestures. Unlike the treatments used in most fads (e.g., bleeding, purging, mercury poisoning),
the dance frenzy may have had beneficial effects mediated by the vig-
orous physical exercise, catharsis, distraction, and group cohesion.

Tarantism and Saint Vitus's dance persisted for four hundred years, from about 1300 to 1700, and then disappeared, with only sporadic cases reported since. This "little ice age" was a difficult time to be alive, with recurrent cycles of famine, pestilence, war, and brigandage. The dancing fads may have offered a cause and a cure for both individual psychopathology and the rampant social breakdown.[3]

Vampire Hysteria (Circa: 1720 to 1770)

The fear of vampires goes far back in time and deep into the human psyche. We have always faced a fundamental problem: what to do with the dead and how to understand what has happened to them. Every culture finds its own solution to this most existential of questions— elaborate burial rituals and folkloric theories are developed to manage the possibly permeable boundary between life and death.

The problem gained poignancy when nomadic hunters and gatherers settled down to farm and began to live quite literally on top of their dead. Previously, corpses were conveniently left behind when the tribe moved on. But forced proximity to dead ancestors gave rise to fear and worship of them. If someone got sick, if something went wrong, it made sense to worry that the dead (who were living underfoot and perhaps feeling envious or vengeful or dissatisfied) might rise up to exact their pound of flesh.

In vampirism, this was believed literally—illness in the living was attributed to the blood drinking or flesh eating of the (not so) departed (not so loving) former loved one. The fad started and ended in central Europe during a fifty-year period in the eighteenth century. The surface intellectual calm of the Age of Enlightenment was a thin veneer covering the raging superstition of turbulent, barely postfeudal, mostly rural Europe. Vampirism emerged when Slavic folktales of the "undead" were carried by word of mouth to new neighbors in the expanding Austrian empire. Dedicated, but credulous, Hapsburg officials made the mistake of being too bureaucratic. Following the methods recommended by their Serbian advisers, they made diligent investigations, conducted exhumations, and dutifully staked corpses. Careful reports detailing the best local practices used in executing vampires were widely circulated. Thus legitimized, terror of the "undead" spread like wildfire from village to village. Soon the writers got into the act and invented a lurid vampire literature that fed the flames and precipitated a frenzy of sightings. Alleged "attacks" were reported in East Prussia in 1721 and throughout the Austrian empire during the 1720s and 1730s. The word *vampire* first entered the English language in 1734, introduced by a travelogue on central Europe. This was the first media-driven fad in history, but not the last.

Vampire worries were heightened by the difficulty of distinguishing between the quick and the dead. Until fairly recently, a lack of medical technology made this a matter of guesswork and dispute. In a world without stethoscopes, there was no clear boundary. People feared the "undead" and also the risk of themselves being buried alive. Graveside vigils were common—not only to show respect, but also to detect renewed signs of life and to discourage grave robbers. The close observation of corpses contributed to legends of their continued appetites and prowess. Corpses vary dramatically in their rates and style of decomposition. People may temporarily look better dead than they ever did alive—the wasted living body more pleasing to the eye when filled out by the gases of decomposition. The ruddy dusky color might suggest the corpse had enjoyed the blood of the living. This logical enough suspicion would be confirmed if blood was seen seeping from the mouth or nose of the undead.

Efforts to extirpate the vampires were unkind to the living and to the dead. For vampires captured on the hoof, there were public executions preceded by tortures of the cruelest kind. The victims were the usual cast of suspects—the mentally ill and mentally challenged; the presumed witches (probably women good with herbs); the suicidal, who flirted with death; rebels from church doctrine; and anyone who might be at the wrong place at the wrong time or have the wrong enemy.

The cure to this craziness came in the person of Maria Theresa, the wise queen of Austria. Her court physician did a thorough study to determine whether vampires actually existed and concluded that there was no basis for any of the claims. The empress then outlawed exhumation under severe penalty, and vampirism died off.

Small, isolated epidemics of vampirism do sometimes still arise—in recent decades, in Puerto Rico, Haiti, Mexico, Malawi, and of all places, London.[4]

Werther Fever Creates Epidemics of Suicide (First Occurrence 1774, and in Flurries Since)

History presents no clearer testimony to the power of great literature (or the danger of fads) than the deadly effect of Goethe's novel *The Sorrows of Young Werther*, published in 1774.[5] This partly autobiographical tale of unrequited love and romantic suicide created a new phenomenon—the author as celebrity, the book as fashion guide. A contagion of Werther fever infected Europe, influencing dress, speech, and manners and provoking a fatal chain of copycat suicides. Ironically, Goethe overcame his own lovesickness, lived into ripe old age, renounced the book, and regretted the harms it had caused. His older and wiser hero, Faust, forsakes the temptations of fickle romance for the safer pleasures of building dikes in Holland.

Imitative suicide has two quite different patterns—cluster and mass. Suicide clusters occur when people copy either a celebrity suicide or that of a relative, friend, classmate, or coworker. Fears of suicide contagion are real enough to have prompted the Centers for Disease Control to issue a set of guidelines on media reporting—suggesting concise, factual stories that avoid glorifying sensationalism, glamorous romance, detailed how-to descriptions, promoting fame by suicide, or any suggestion that suicide can be a rational choice or a gateway to lasting fame.[6]

Mass suicide has a socially sanctioned motivation. There have been dozens of episodes throughout history of defeated armies (or their women and children) committing suicide together rather than face murder or enslavement. Less frequent is the protest suicide, when a group jointly decides to make their point in the strongest possible way. A third variant is the group suicide (kamikaze) mission in defense of a religion, ideal, or nation. Then there are the mass religious suicides: follow-the-leader behavior commanded by some would-be messiah.

Natural selection has been ruthless and largely successful in pruning out suicidal DNA. Despite all of life's vicissitudes, only one in a thousand people take death into their own hands. The self-destructive often die young, taking their genes with them into oblivion. Life-affirming DNA wins the procreation sweepstakes and keeps us struggling to stay in the game, whatever the hardship and pain. In suicide epidemics, the herd instinct overwhelms our powerful instinct for self-preservation. There is no better illustration of the countervailing power of fads than the fact that the urge to join one sometimes trumps staying alive.

vicissitudes = downturns, changes

Neuroscience Promotes Clinical Fads

Neurasthenia, hysteria, and multiple personality disorder were three late-nineteenth-century fads all started by charismatic neurologists (Beard and Charcot) to explain the puzzlingly, nonspecific presentations of many of their patients. Why three epidemics all at once? And why all three started by neurologists? This is a cautionary (and currently very relevant) tale of how the brilliance of neuroscience findings can sometimes give undeserved authority to half-cocked clinical ideas. The conditions then were similar to conditions now: there was a revolution in understanding how the brain works. The neuron had just been discovered, and scientists (including Freud) were busy tracing the paths of its complex web of synaptic connections. The brain was revealed to be an electrical machine, much more complex but not fundamentally different from the many new electrical devices just then being invented and entering the mainstream of daily life.

The new biology of brain would explain behaviors previously considered to be within the abstract provinces of the philosophers and the theologians. It might be impossible to plumb the depths of the human soul, but it should be possible to figure out the structural specifications and electrical connections of the human brain. Symptoms were not the result of demonic possession, curse, sin, vampires, or tarantula bites. They were understandable as malfunctions in the wiring of the brain machine. This was, and is, a powerful and accurate model. But (then as now) the problem was underestimating just how difficult it is to probe the secrets of this remarkably complex machine. The authority of compelling neuroscience gave undeserved dignity to daffy clinical concepts that don't make much sense.

Thus were born the three fads "neurasthenia," "hysteria," and "multiple personality." Each was a different way of labeling and pretending to understand otherwise confusingly nonspecific human suffering. None turned out to be useful; in some ways all were harmful. Their causal explanations were wrong and the treatment recommendations at best had the efficacy of placebo and more often worsened the problems they were meant to cure. But the labels flourished for decades because they sounded convincing, stood on the high authority of the emerging science of neurology, were promoted by charismatic thought leaders, and met the human need for explanation. This all sounds very current and provides an important lesson. A powerfully convincing, but incorrect and harmful, set of labels and causal theories fooled the smartest doctors and the smartest patients in the world. These were revolutionary best guesses that turned out to be dead wrong—as will many of ours.

Neurasthenia (Circa Late 1800s to Early 1900s)

Starting in 1869, an American neurologist named George Miller Beard defined and successfully promoted neurasthenia—literally, weak nerves. He was attempting to fill a diagnostic black hole—how to label the many people with the nonspecific bodily and psychological symptoms of fatigue, loss of energy, weakness, dizziness, fainting, dyslexia, flatulence, headache, generalized aches and pains, trouble sleeping, and impotence; depression or anxiety or both. Neurasthenia had the attraction of seeming to explain this wide waterfront of commonplace symptoms.

Beard's causal theory followed a hydraulics model analogous to a power failure in any electrical machine—physical and mental exhaustion was plausibly linked to a depletion of the central nervous system's energy supply. Beard attributed this depletion to social causes—how hard it was for people to adjust to a rapidly changing technological civilization, the stresses of urbanization, and the increasingly competitive business environment. People were getting sick because they were pushing themselves beyond their tolerance and reserves. Most cases occurred in the striving classes of sedentary workers—because they were tiring their minds when nature meant them to be tiring their bodies. Sigmund Freud, then a neurologist, accepted the usefulness of neurasthenia as a descriptive diagnosis because it so well described many of his patients. But he developed a completely different theory to explain the energy depletion—depleted libido. This could be constitutional or result from having too many orgasms (most often from excessive masturbation).

The treatments for neurasthenia have been remarkably varied, nonspecific, and silly. Beard's preferred treatment was a biological juice-up of the system with electrotherapy. Freud mocked this as "pretense treatment" and instead suggested a reduction of libidinal depleting activities like masturbation or excessive intercourse. He did not recommend psychoanalysis for neurasthenia because it was caused by libidinal deficit, not psychological conflict. Treatments suggested by others included rest cures, bathing cures, dietary changes, and distraction from the cares of everyday life. All probably had at best the impact of a good placebo.

Neurasthenia was a vague and nondescript diagnosis with vague, nondescript, and useless treatments. That this did not reduce its enormous worldwide popularity should tell us a great deal about the seductiveness of clinical confabulations. We have an intellectual need to find an elephant in the cloud. The label we create, however inaccurate, provides a comforting explanation of the patient's suffering and a target for treatment. It is a metaphor of distress appropriate to the technology and worldview of a particular time and place. When everyone is interested in electrical power, the metaphor of distress becomes energy depletion. When people get interested in neurotransmitters (as is the case now), the glib metaphor becomes "chemical imbalance."

Neurasthenia disappeared suddenly—probably because psychiatrists replaced neurologists as the major caregivers of patients with nonspecific and vague physical and mental symptoms. The switch from neurology to psychiatry occasioned a parallel switch from physical to psychological symptoms as the preferred mode of communication between patient and doctor. The psychiatric nomenclature was also expanding and soon became much more specific in describing a wide variety of different outpatient presentations that were previously lumped under the unifying, but essentially meaningless, label of neurasthenia. The fad had run its course.[7]

Hysteria/Conversion Disorder (Circa Late 1800s to Early 1900s)

Of all epidemics, this one had the highest pedigree, promoted as it was by the four most famous neurologists of the time—Jean-Martin

Charcot, Pierre-Marie-Félix Janet, Josef Breuer, and Freud. Hysteria described patients presenting with neurological symptoms that were puzzling because they did not conform to the distribution of the nervous system or to established neurological disease. Most common were paralysis, sensory loss, strange sensations, posturing, speech loss or alteration, gagging, convulsions, dizziness, or loss of consciousness.

Charcot was a great showman who addressed hysteria with an enthusiasm and flair that should have set off alarms. He gathered a stable of highly suggestible patients and an army of students (including Freud) who came to Paris from all of Europe to see the master at work in demonstrations that were well attended, highly dramatic, and photogenic. Charcot reveled in proving that hypnosis could both cure and create the symptoms—he could hypnotize the halt and the lame and make them well; or he could hypnotize the well and make them halt and lame. His patients, many of them housed together, became wonderful mimics of one another's symptoms even when outside the auspices of the great man. Somehow, Charcot missed the central point of all this. His power of suggestion and the effort to please him had turned his patients into performers, just as he had also become one. Not recognizing his own causative role, Charcot evolved vague theories of brain disease that presumably made one susceptible to both hypnosis and to hysteria.

Meanwhile, back in Vienna, Breuer (Freud's other teacher) was having trouble hypnotizing Anna O. She was a creative, intelligent, suggestible, and lonely woman with the usual panoply of nonspecific, mostly neurological symptoms. Under her guidance, the "talking cure" (or psychoanalysis) was invented as an alternative to hypnosis. Instead of going into a hypnotic trance, Anna associated seemingly random thoughts. Then patient and doctor made psychological connections linking her fantasies and unconscious impulses to her past life. It worked! Symptoms promptly improved. But Anna would get sick again whenever her recovery threatened to end the cherished relationship with Breuer. There was an obvious explanation. Anna got better to please Breuer and got worse to avoid losing him. This made Breuer nervous (to say nothing of his jealous wife, who probably understood Anna's motives a lot more clearly than he or Freud ever did).

It was clear, as with Charcot's hypnosis, that symptoms could be made to disappear or to appear based on the patient's suggestibility and that suggestion was an important force in every powerful doctor-patient relationship. Freud coined the term "transference" for the parental role that tied patients to their doctors and made them so vulnerable to influence. But Freud failed to understand how big a role suggestion also plays in psychoanalysis. He understood and overvalued intrapsychic conflict and transference; he failed to understand and undervalued the current interpersonal relationship.[8]

Psychoanalysis was an ineffective treatment for conversion disorder and, like hypnosis, contributed to propagating it. Ironically, a shaman would be a more effective therapist for Anna O. than a psychoanalyst. He would understand her symptom as metaphor and would find a more effective way of suggesting it away. The treatment of Anna O. ended badly, with Anna still sick and angry at Breuer. But there was a happy ending. In real life, Anna O. was Bertha Pappenheim, who recovered and went on to become one of the founders of the profession of social work.

As with neurasthenia, conversion hysteria disappeared when psychiatrists replaced neurologists as the primary caregivers for this population of help seekers. Suggestible patients seeing neurologists naturally enough presented with neurological symptoms. The same patient seeing a psychoanalyst would express suffering with more emotional and cognitive symptoms. Conversion symptoms continue to be seen in parts of the world where there are few mental health workers and patients can best access help through physical symptoms.[9]

Multiple Personality Disorder

Multiple personality disorder first became common in Europe at the turn of the twentieth century. Charcot was again the pied piper. He had helped to make hypnosis a popular medical treatment (when it wasn't also doubling as a popular parlor trick). The hypnotic trance brought to light unacceptable feelings, fantasies, memories, and urges previously kept outside conscious awareness. A collaboration of suggestible patients and suggestible doctors elaborated the notion that the individual was harboring a hidden personality (or two or three or more). Through a process of "dissociation," the hidden personalities had established their own independent existence and might even at times temporarily take charge and do things that were outside the control, or even the awareness, of the dominant personality. This was a way of converting a metaphor of distress and discomfort with oneself into a seemingly coherent disease that would also reduce any personal responsibility for the disowned feelings.

Paradoxically, the way to treat the dissociation that presumably caused the multiplication of personality was to encourage even more dissociation through hypnosis. The goal was to induce the "alter" personalities to enter the light of day so that they might be melded together into a cohesive whole. Not surprisingly, the overall effect of hypnotic treatment was to promote, rather than to cure, the presumed illness—the submerged personalities continued to divide and multiply. Fortunately, therapists and patients eventually caught on that hypnosis was doing more harm than good, and it became less popular. Multiple personality disorder disappeared when hypnotists were replaced by psychoanalysts, who focused the patient's attention on fragmented repressed impulses and memories, rather than on integrating repressed personalities.

There was a brief resurgence of multiple personality in the mid-1950s suggested by the popular book and movie *The Three Faces of*

Eve.[10] It didn't last long because most therapists were analytically trained and uninterested in multiple personality disorder. There was no cadre of therapists ready, willing, and able to create a cadre of new MPD patients. A more enduring fad followed after *Sybil* in the 1970s. The volume of MPD cases began rising dramatically; the fad fed on itself, peaked in the early 1990s, and then disappeared as suddenly as it had emerged. The revival of MPD was fueled by a renewed therapeutic interest in hypnosis and other regressive and suggestive treatments aimed at bringing out "alters." An industry of therapists was born during weekend workshops where they learned how best to uncover new personalities. This poorly trained army of enthusiastic newly branded MPD "experts" created new personalities at an alarming clip, and MPD became the default "diagnosis du jour" for every patient seen in their practice.

MPD is probably no more than a metaphor that has taken on a life of its own. Most (if not all) of the MPD cases were induced by the efforts of these well-meaning but misguided therapists who were as clueless about what was going on as were the patients. It is not hard for a suggestible therapist treating a suggestible patient to turn any run-of-the-mill psychiatric problem into MPD. The individual and the doctor conjure up and name the "alter(s)" to give coherence to fragmentary and unacceptable impulses and behaviors that are in conflict with self-expectations. It is not a far step to assume they have an independent existence.[11]

For a while it seemed that every third or fourth patient was claiming to have multiple personalities. The fad was also fed by the Internet's (then emerging) ability to provide instant information and support. As the number of people with MPD grew, so did the number of personalities per person, and a competition developed to determine who could achieve the most "alters." The record in my experience was set by a woman who claimed to have unearthed 162 distinct personalities (mostly female but including a couple of dozen males), of widely varying ages and dispositions, and each with a name. The whole thing got even sillier when some patients (and even, believe it or not, some therapists) began to assert that the multiple personalities were somehow related to demonic possession and satanic rituals.

The demand for MPD treatment dropped dramatically when insurance stopped paying for it and when therapists grew fatigued and disillusioned. MPD enthusiasts came to realize they were opening a Pandora's box by inducing more and more personalities. The patients usually got progressively worse, sometimes much worse, and were difficult to handle in treatment and in life. I have seen at least a hundred people who claimed to harbor multiple personalities. Almost all of them presented in a flock during the heyday of the epidemic in the late 1980s and early 1990s. In every case, I discovered that the emerging personalities had taken on a life of their own only after the patient had entered treatment with a psychotherapist interested in the topic, or after joining an Internet chat group, or after meeting someone else with the problem, or after seeing a movie that portrayed it. I wonder if MPD ever occurs as a spontaneous clinical entity—if so, it cannot be very often.

MPD presented a dilemma for me in my work as chair of the *DSM-IV* Task Force. I felt it was a hoax (or more kindly a collective temporary contagion of therapist and patient suggestibility) and certainly not a legitimate mental disorder. For better and worse, I chose not to impose my view on *DSM-IV*. We continue to include MPD in the manual and we took scrupulous pains to present both sides of the controversy as fairly and effectively as possible—even though I believed one side was complete bunk. I was hoisted on my own conservative petard—not to make changes based only on my own opinion. Thankfully, the world has taken a break and for now has moved away from MPD, but I would expect other outbreaks in the future. Multiple personality seems to have an enduring appeal to suggestible patients and suggestible therapists and lies dormant, ready to make a comeback. We are always just a blockbuster movie and some weekend therapist's workshops away from a new fad. Look for another epidemic beginning in a decade or two as a new generation of therapists forgets the lessons of the past.

What about MPD makes frances believe it will revive again in the future?

Witch Hunts: The Day Care Sex Abuse Scandal (Circa 1980 to 2000)

vitriolic: cruel & bitter criticism
prurient: encouraging an excessive interest in sexual matters

The day care sex scandals (occurring contemporaneously with, and sometimes related to, the MPD fad) were a close replay of the Salem witch trials. Separated by exactly three hundred years, both epidemics reflect the worst in human nature and were fueled by the same ingredients of fear, vitriolic accusation, prurient puritanism, suggestion, projection, group contagion, and the credulous acceptance of the obviously fantastic testimony of children. The Salem witch hunts of the 1690s were propagated by righteous (but misguided and destructive) Puritan ministers. In the United States in the 1990s, the epidemic was fostered by well-meaning (but misguided and destructive) therapists—admittedly ably assisted by misguided parents, police, prosecutors, judges, and juries. This is a discouraging tale, an outrageous miscarriage of justice, and a discouraging breakdown in our civil society.

The cases all followed the same depressing script. The fad began in Kern County, California, in 1982 and, within ten years, had spread like wildfire across the country (and to a lesser degree around the world). There were allegations that day care workers were sexually abusing their charges, often in the most shocking and bizarre ways. In every case, the evidence was based on wild and fantastic accusations made by very young children, unsupported by physical evidence or credible corroborative testimony. The initial charge would usually be made by a vindictive or deranged accuser—usually a parent, stepparent, or grandparent. The panic would soon spread to other parents and the community at large.

The testimony of the children was a confabulation derived from long, repeated, and grueling inquisitions conducted by an unholy alliance of therapists, police officers, and prosecutors—egged on by parents and press. The tone of the interrogators was leading, suggestive, and at times even coercive. They already knew what terrible things had happened—it was just a question of having the child victims fill in the gory details. The kids were told what the other kids were saying and great pressure was applied to get them to conform and confirm. The stories offered by the different child witnesses naturally fed on one another and gradually converged into a seemingly consistent and damning picture. Salem redux.

There was no shortage of lurid, ready-made details to fill in any holes in the child's imagination or recollection of events. The possible limitations of creativity of a given interviewer or child were supplemented by wide and wild media reporting of the charges that had been made in other cases. The press and TV were having a field day and providing a circus. That the charges were ridiculous, fantastic, and physically impossible did not matter. One would assume that no reasonable person could possibly grant them any credibility, but people had stopped being reasonable. The weirdest accusations gained a crazy authority if they were repeated enough in any given case. And they seemed to confirm what had been reported so often and so loudly and with such vivid detail in so many different cases in so many different states and countries. There had to be fire, since there was so much smoke. The judicial system could cop a plea to its own temporary insanity.

The cases played different variations on two themes of abuse—sexual and satanic. The sexual part consisted of every imaginable sex act (and some that are not imaginable or even possible) and of orgies, pornography, prostitution, and torture. The satanic rites consisted of devil worship, killing or torturing animals, drinking blood or urine, eating feces, and demonic possession. Some of the stories contained obviously fantastic elements—alien contact, abuse by robots, knife stabbings that left no wounds, and so on. The patent absurdity of some of these claims somehow failed to alert the eager pursuers to the likely absurdity of all of them.

All these horrible goings-on would purportedly occur at the day care center during its regularly appointed hours with no one noticing—not parents, or neighbors, or delivery men, no one. It went unexplained how, up to the point of exposure of the foul deeds, the children could leave the center each day smiling and normal. Things got worse as the methods of grand inquisition ground into gear. The suspicion and blame spread. Clearly the primary perpetrator could not have gone undetected in his corrupting acts without the conspiratorial connivance or active participation of the entire staff of the day care center. These poor innocent souls would be subjected to the righteous wrath and brutal interrogation techniques of naive (but often ambitious) public servants determined to protect our children and to punish severely all those responsible for their lost innocence. The coworkers faced the usual horrible choice of those who have been accused unfairly—lose honor or lose freedom. Confess to false charges that they had participated in the absurd activities alleged by their child accusers, thus betraying their friends who will be found guilty based on their false testimony. Or face a long prison term for the crime of having been innocently in the wrong place at the wrong time.

In a panicked and frenzied desire to protect their children from an imagined loss of innocence, the parents subjected them to damaging interrogation, fantastic concepts about sex and Satan, the need to lie and bear false witness, public exposure, and later guilt for being part of this mess. Certainly they caused their children to have a real loss of innocence. The "therapists" involved in the cases had developed an instant expertise on day care sex and would soon acquire celebrity for their heroic efforts to root it out. The interviewers were remarkably blind to the effect of their biases and the role of suggestion and positive reinforcement in helping to get the children to parrot their preconceptions. The therapists furthered the process by using anatomically correct dolls, presumably for an evidentiary purpose to determine what had actually occurred. But it degenerated instead into a mutual play therapy that elicited ever more fantastic fantasies from the collaborative sexual imaginations of the children and the therapists.[12]

Why did the epidemic of day care hysteria happen just when and where it did? Why in 1982? Why in the United States? It is never possible to be precise in evaluating the causes of any event that has so many different and interacting influences. But some things stand out as likely contributors. You can't have a panic about day care centers unless you have day care centers. These had become a necessary fixture of American life as more mothers entered the workforce, families traveled far distances to chase available jobs, and there were fewer available grandmothers to help babysit. Undoubtedly parental guilt in turning over parental responsibility played a role. Among therapists, there was concern over previously not taking seriously enough the statements of kids who had actually experienced sexual abuse. There were also too many therapists with too little expertise who were able nonetheless to self-promote and gain authority as fake "experts." This sad episode is the clearest caution imaginable to any therapist feeling the impulse to jump onto a current or future fad bandwagon.

Following the Pack

We should not be surprised that psychiatric diagnosis has always been, and still is, so faddish. Fashion influences every aspect of our behavior, and following the pack is part of human nature. The good news is that fashions come and fashions go. A century ago, the world was awash in neurasthenia, conversion hysteria, and multiple personality disorder. Then all three suddenly and mysteriously disappeared. The psychiatric fads that now seem so entrenched are less robust than meets the eye and will likely also wilt with time and as people come to understand their risks. But there's also bad news. Most epidemics in the past were isolated, local, and self-limited. Our new fads are globalized, monetized, and becoming part of the societal infrastructure.

CHAPTER 5

Fads of the Present

"When I use a word," Humpty Dumpty said, in a rather scornful tone, "it means just what I choose it to mean— neither more nor less."
"The question is," said Alice, "whether you can make words mean so many different things."
"The question is," said Humpty Dumpty, "which is to be master—that's all."
LEWIS CARROLL, *Alice's Adventures in Wonderland*

HUMPTY DUMPTY BRAGS unrealistically about his ability to master words and control their definition. His pride qualifies him for the well-deserved great fall he is about to have. One of the things Alice is constantly discovering in Wonderland is that words can fly out of control and have different and confusing meanings, very dependent on context. It is not so much what you "choose to mean" as it is what others take you to mean. And that can be much more or much less than you intended.

We were unaware how much we were in Humpty's precarious position when *DSM-IV* was published in 1994. We shared his complacent belief in the power of carefully chosen words and were surprised when ours also flew out of control. Our goal was to prevent diagnostic inflation from growing and our conceit was to think we had succeeded in holding the line.[1] We were wrong.[2] It turns out that the impact of the diagnostic system is not in the words as written, it's in the way words come to be used. *DSM-IV* was meant to be a careful and conservative diagnostic manual, but once out of our hands, it was not always used carefully and conservatively. We thought we shot down every new suggestion that might be a giveaway to the drug industry. But we greatly underestimated their power to convince practitioners and patients to apply our words in the loosest possible way. A colorful TV commercial has much more dramatic impact than the fine print of a dry *DSM-IV* criteria set. The constant blitz of misleading marketing easily overwhelmed the barriers to overdiagnosis we thought were built into our definitions. As it turned out, *DSM-IV* unwittingly contributed to three new false epidemics in psychiatry—the overdiagnosis of attention deficit, autism, and adult bipolar disorder. Rule of thumb—if anything in a *DSM* can possibly be misused, it will be misused.

We should have known better. Conflicts between the written and oral tradition are as old as the Bible and as current as the Supreme Court's interpretation of the Constitution. The written words themselves generally don't rule—it is all in their later interpretation. Alternate productions of the same play can each convey very different meanings without ever changing one single word. The lesson of the last fifteen years is that the *DSM* alone does not establish standards. Physicians, other mental health workers, drug companies, advocacy groups, school systems, the courts, the Internet, and cable TV all get to vote on how the written word will actually be used and misused. There are false prophets and false epidemics. You get to exert control over the diagnostic manual only up to the moment you publish it. Once it is out in the public domain, people use it (and often misuse it) as they damn well please.

Below is a rogues' gallery of the current false epidemics in psychiatry—

the mental disorders most likely to be overdiagnosed and overtreated. Describing them will hopefully reduce their spread. But first, one important caveat—a fad diagnosis is a useful diagnosis gone wild. Many, perhaps most of the people who currently have the diagnosis have gotten it for good reason. These are "fads" only because they have become too fashionable and are often loosely and inappropriately applied—particularly in primary care. Each, in its right place and accurately diagnosed, is absolutely essential to understanding and treating psychiatric symptoms. Anyone at the margins who has already received one of these diagnoses should get a second opinion. Always be skeptical, but not too skeptical.

Attention Deficit Disorder Runs Wild

It is 6:00 A.M., dark and rainy, and I am driving to the airport. I can't put up the top to my convertible because it has been broken for months, but I keep forgetting to get it fixed. I arrive, double-park to check my bags, leaving the lights on and the radio blaring golden oldies from the 1960s, 1970s, and 1980s. On returning a week later, I can't find my car in the garage. This is surprising to me, but shouldn't be, because I never parked it there. I forgot it altogether, just checked the bags and blithely boarded the plane. Good-humored security officers call in all their buddies to enjoy a hearty laugh at my expense. I am enormously grateful to them for towing my car to a safe place, charging my battery, and refusing any money because the rare experience of meeting anyone so silly has been more than enough reward.

My secretary, Tammy, has similarly found her life enriched by the delectation of my magical ability to lose papers going the ten feet from her office to mine, my repeated inability to find my office in a hospital maze I have worked in for years, and my capacity to forget meetings and appointments. My wife is much less connoisseur than critic. She unempathically claims that my lack of attention to the needs and errands of everyday life reflects willful avoidance rather than diagnosable mental disorder. My life has been a kind of sheltered workshop. The kindness of friends and strangers has protected me from any serious impairment.

Am I an absentminded professor or psychiatrically sick? Should I start taking stimulants or muddle through after my fashion? In the old days I was a normal, if sometimes ridiculous, person. But things are different now. ADHD is spreading like wildfire. It used to be confined to a small percentage of kids who had clear-cut problems that started at a very early age and caused them unmistakable difficulties in many situations. Then all manner of classroom disruption was medicalized and ADHD was applied so promiscuously that an amazing 10 percent of kids now qualify. Every classroom now has at least one or two kids on medication. And increasingly, ADHD is becoming an explain-all for all sorts of performance problems in adults as well.

How could this possibly happen? There were six contributors: wording changes in *DSM-IV*; heavy drug company marketing to doctors and advertising to the general public; extensive media coverage; pressure from harried parents and teachers to control unruly children; extra time given on tests and extra school services for those with an ADHD diagnosis; and finally, the widespread misuse of prescription stimulants for general performance enhancement and recreation.

The most obvious explanation is by far the least likely—that the real prevalence of attentional and hyperactivity problems has actually increased. There is no reason to think the kids have changed, it is just that the labels have. We now diagnose as mental disorder attentional and behavioral problems that used to be seen as part of life and of normal individual variation. The most convincing evidence of this comes from a large study with a particularly disturbing finding. A child's date of birth was a very powerful predictor of whether or not he would get the diagnosis of ADHD. Boys born in January were at 70 percent higher risk than those born in December simply because January 1 was the cutoff for grade assignment. The youngest, least developmentally mature kids in the class are much more likely to get the

ADHD diagnosis. The birthday effect was almost as influential in girls. We have turned being immature because of being young into a disease to be treated with a pill.[3,4,5]

The *DSM-IV* contribution was inadvertent and probably only a bit player in the selling of ADHD. We changed a few words so that the definition would be more female friendly—taking into account that girls are more likely to be inattentive "space cadets" and less likely than boys to be hyperactive. Extensive field testing predicted only a 15 percent increase in rates, but we were later blindsided by clever drug marketing which caused rates to triple. Until the mid-1990s, ADHD had occupied a tiny, sleepy corner of the vast and active pharmaceutical enterprise, barely worth noting. The stimulant drugs used to treat ADHD had been off patent for decades and could be purchased in generic form for pennies a pill. Total revenues of $50 million a year for ADHD medications amounted to no more than a rounding error in drug company financial reports. There was no advertising to patients or marketing to doctors. ADHD seemed a safe, no-profit diagnosis flying well under Pharma's searching radar.

Conditions changed dramatically a few years after the publication of *DSM-IV*. Several newly patented and expensive ADHD medications came on the market. Coincidentally, the drug companies had just been given the right to advertise to consumers—and did they ever take advantage of this with an all-media-all-the-time advertising fanfare. The blaring propaganda message was the usual—ADHD is extremely common, often missed, and accounts for why Johnny is a behavioral problem and isn't learning in school. "Ask your doctor." Armies of eager sales reps filled the offices of pediatricians, family doctors, and psychiatrists peddling a pill that would magically prevent classroom disruptions and solve home meltdowns. Parents, teachers, and physicians were recruited in an all-out effort to identify and aggressively treat ADHD.[6,7]

There is lingering controversy on how much the tripled prevalence of ADHD should be the cause of celebration or serious concern or perhaps both. Some believe that the higher rates mostly reflect the useful identification of ADHD in people who were previously missed. This is partly true. No doubt increased diagnosis has been helpful for many children who otherwise would not have received a much-needed and appropriate treatment. Medication for these correctly diagnosed kids can (at least in the short run) improve learning, prevent restlessness, reduce impulsive outbursts, help them feel more comfortable in their own skins, and reduce blame and stigma. For children who really need it, stimulant medication is safe and effective—a real godsend to them, their parents, and teachers.

But there is an unhappy flip side to this feel-good story. The gains to some have to be offset against the serious costs to others. Much of the increased prevalence of ADHD results from the "false positive" misidentification of kids who would be better off never receiving a diagnosis. Drug company marketing pressure often leads to unnecessary treatment with medications that can cause the harmful side effects of insomnia, loss of appetite, irritability, heart rhythm problems, and a variety of psychiatric symptoms. Add to this the emerging problem of stimulant misuse for performance enhancement and intoxication. Do we really want 30 percent of our college students and 10 percent of our high school students scoring prescription stimulants illegally so they can do better on a test or have more fun at a party? Monitoring the large, illegal secondary street and school market for stimulant drugs has even made it hard to have adequate supplies for legitimate purposes.[8]

How can we cut down on loose diagnosis and excessive use of medication? Just a few doctors in each community are responsible for most of the overprescribing. Quality controls and shaming can dramatically tame their practice habits.[9] Doctors also need education that, contrary to what they have learned from Pharma, the best approach to ADHD is a graduated "stepped diagnosis"—not "shoot first, aim later." Diagnose early and begin medication quickly only when the ADHD symptoms are very severe, pressingly urgent, and classic in presentation. Whenever symptoms are mild or equivocal (as often is the case), it is best to sit back and have a period of watchful waiting. Often the symptoms will be transient—reactive to family, peer, or school stress. Sometimes the kid is just immature. Sometimes the problem is substance abuse or another psychiatric disorder that needs to be ruled out during the period of observation. If the problems persist but are not severely impairing, the next steps would be educational or psychotherapeutic in orientation. The final step of definitive diagnosis and medication treatment would be reserved only for those who fail to respond adequately to earlier steps. Unfortunately, there is no well-financed public and physician educational campaign to promote this sensible stepped approach. The drug company rush-to-diagnosis and mindlessly prescribe-the-pill message has dominated the conversation—turning many normally immature kids into prematurely medicated mental patients.

Childhood Bipolar Disorder

When I began psychiatric training forty-five years ago, we were not taught anything about childhood bipolar disorder (CBD). There was no point—it was so vanishingly rare that no one had seen any cases. I once evaluated a nine-year-old boy whose symptoms seemed bipolar, but my supervisor told me to stop searching for the exotic. His advice was "when you hear hoofbeats on Broadway, assume it's horses out there, not zebras." In those old days, we were undoubtedly missing some cases of childhood bipolar and sometimes withholding what might have been helpful treatment.

But now the pendulum has swung wildly and dangerously in the other direction. CBD has become the most inflated bubble in all of psychiatric diagnosis, with a remarkable fortyfold inflation in just one decade. CBD satisfied three essential preconditions for excessive popularity: a pressing need, influential prophets, and an engaging story.

The pressing need was created by the disturbed and disturbing kids encountered in clinical, school, and correctional settings. They suffer and cause suffering to those around them—making themselves noticeable to families, doctors, and teachers. Everyone feels enormous pressure to do something. Previous diagnoses (especially conduct or oppositional disorder) provided little hope and no call to action. In contrast, a diagnosis of CBD purports (falsely) to explain the misbehavior and justifies a medication intervention.

The false prophets were influential and charismatic "thought leaders" who had the added prestige of coming from Harvard. They spread an apocryphal gospel evangelized widely to child psychiatrists, pediatricians, family physicians, parents, and teachers. Their energetic crusade was heavily financed by the drug company sponsors who would be the major beneficiaries. The prophets had gone up to the mountaintop and come down with a new dogma—henceforth the old *DSM* rules for diagnosing bipolar need not apply to children. CBD no longer required the presence of classic mood swings between mania and depression. Instead the diagnosis could be made in a free-form, inclusive way to include a variegated hodgepodge of kids who were irritable, temperamental, angry, aggressive, and/or impulsive. The CBD boundaries were thus to be pushed far into unfamiliar territory to label children who previously received other diagnoses (e.g., attention deficit, conduct, oppositional, or anxiety disorder) or no diagnosis at all ("temperamental" but normal kids). A vast new market was opened for grateful Pharma. Mood swings are rare in kids—not a good sales target. But irritability is common enough to bring in blockbuster sales. And bipolar disorder is usually considered a lifelong diagnosis. Turn a child of tender age into a customer and he might be yours for life.

It is not at all surprising that the pharmaceutical industry pushed the expanded definition of CBD and cashed in on its newfound popularity. More surprising was the enthusiastic acquiescence of doctors, therapists, parents, teachers, advocacy groups, the media, and the Internet.

Once the rigors of *DSM-IV* definition were thrown out the window, mood-stabilizing and antipsychotic medications were given out wildly to treat fake CBD. The results have been devastating. Kids can have a rapid and substantial weight gain—an average twelve pounds in twelve weeks—increasing the risk of diabetes and possibly reducing life span.[10,11,12] The most egregious malpractice has been loading up two- and three-year-olds with medication to treat a ridiculously premature diagnosis of bipolar disorder—in some cases killing them with lethal overdoses.[13]

CBD also carries considerable stigma, implying that the child will have a lifelong illness requiring lifetime treatment. The diagnosis can distort a person's life narrative, cutting off hopes of otherwise achievable ambitions, and also may reduce a sense of control over, and responsibility for, undesirable behavior. Other more specific causes of temper outbursts are much shorter lived and amenable to time-limited treatment. Substance abuse should always be the first thought for any irritable teenager. And attention deficit disorder often presents with an irritability that responds best to stimulants, but these may be withheld in the face of an incorrect bipolar diagnosis.

The CBD fad is the most shameful episode in my forty-five years of observing psychiatry. The widespread use of dangerous medicine to treat a fake diagnosis constitutes a vast public health experiment with no informed consent.

It is some small comfort that it did not arise from anything we wrote into *DSM-IV*—we rejected the suggestion for a criteria specific to CBD that would have legitimized the fad and given it more force. But I wish we had put a black box warning in the bipolar disorder section cautioning clinicians not to be fast and loose in giving young kids a diagnosis that most often did not apply to them and could have such dangerous consequences.

Autism Becomes Fashionable

The diagnosis of autism has exploded in the past twenty years. Before *DSM-IV*, this was an extremely rare condition, diagnosed in one child per two thousand. The rate has now jumped to one in eighty in the United States and an even more amazing one in thirty-eight in Korea.[14,15,16] The first reaction was parental panic—worries about autism at the slightest sign that a child was not perfectly conventional. This was reinforced by a paper in *The Lancet* suggesting that autism might be caused by vaccination. In fact, their co-occurrence is no more than a coincidental chronological fluke—the typical age of onset of autism happens to occur at around the same time that vaccinations are scheduled. Conclusive studies have since disproved any causal connection, and *The Lancet* retracted the original paper when it was later exposed as a scientific fraud.[17] But despite all the evidence to the contrary, misplaced parental fear somehow persists. Avoiding vaccination to protect against a false epidemic of autism has put many kids at risk for very real epidemics of measles and other once conquered and sometimes dangerous childhood diseases. All this reflects the general public misunderstanding of how psychiatric diagnosis works—i.e., that the prevalence rates are always extremely sensitive to any change in definition. The twentyfold increase in just twenty years occurred because diagnostic habits had changed radically, not because kids were suddenly becoming more autistic.[18]

The autism "epidemic" has three causes. Some part surely comes from improved surveillance and identification by doctors, teachers, families, and the patients themselves. Spotlighting any problem reduces stigma and improves case finding. Some was triggered by the *DSM-IV* introduction of Asperger's disorder, a new diagnosis that greatly broadened the concept of autism. But about half of the "epidemic" is probably service driven—children get the diagnosis incorrectly because it is the ticket to more attention in the school system and more intense mental health treatment.

Few people have the incapacitating symptoms of classic autism, and these are extremely easy to identify. In contrast, Asperger's describes people who are strange in some ways (with stereotyped interests, unusual behaviors, and interpersonal problems) but not nearly so gravely impaired as those who have classic autism (which also includes an inability to communicate and lowered IQ). Because many normal people are eccentric and socially awkward, there is no clear line of demarcation separating them from Asperger's. We had estimated that Asperger's would be about three times more common than the classic, severe form of autism. But rates have artificially swelled because many people within the range of normal variability (or with other mental disorders) have been misidentified as autistic—especially when the diagnosis is made in primary care, in school systems, and by parents and patients.

DSM-IV may have started the autism epidemic, but other powerful engines drove it forward beyond all expectation. Probably most important was the positive feedback loop between spirited patient advocacy and the provision of school and therapeutic programs that require an autism diagnosis. As the population of "autistic" patients and their families grew, they gained the power to push for many additional services—sometimes by initiating successful lawsuits. The additional services then provided further incentive to increased diagnosis. With more people diagnosed, there was then an even larger constituency to push for more services.[19,20]

The stigma of autism was also greatly reduced. The Internet provided a convenient and comfortable mode of communication, social support, and camaraderie. Autism received extensive and favorable press and television coverage and was presented sympathetically in movies and documentaries. Many successful people recognized themselves in the Asperger's definition, and some wore it as a proud badge. Asperger's even gained its own kind of offbeat glamour, especially among high-tech types. This publicity had the positive effect of reducing the sting of being diagnosed. But there was the usual overshoot. Asperger's went from nowhere to being a diagnosis du jour and explain-all for all sorts of individual difference. About half the kids now diagnosed don't really meet the criteria when these are applied carefully, and about half will have outgrown it on repeat evaluations.[21,22,23,24]

The epidemic has had both pluses and minuses. For correctly identified patients, getting a diagnosis has brought the advantages of improved school and therapeutic services, diminished stigma, increased family understanding, reduced sense of isolation, and Internet support. For mislabeled patients, there are the personal costs of stigma and the reduced self and family expectations. And there is the societal cost of misallocation of extremely scarce and precious resources. It would be better if school decisions were not so closely coupled to a psychiatric diagnosis that was developed originally only for clinical, not at all for educational, purposes. Many of the mislabeled kids do have other serious problems that would independently require them to get special attention; they just don't need the extra added stigma that comes with an incorrect diagnosis of autism. School services should be based on school need, not psychiatric diagnosis.

As chair of the *DSM-IV* Task Force, I deserve blame for not having anticipated the rush to overdiagnose Asperger's. It would have been useful in advance to predict the changes in diagnostic rates and to explain their causes. We should have proactively taken steps to educate the public and the media about what the labels mean and what they don't mean—that the kids hadn't changed, just the way they were being diagnosed. It is a lot easier to trigger a fad than to end one.

Bipolar II

Perhaps the most important distinction in all of psychiatry is unfortunately often the most difficult. Does the patient have bipolar mood swings (with cyclical lows alternating with highs) or is this just a straight unipolar depression (recurrent lows with no highs)? This differential diagnosis has huge implications for future treatment. Antidepressants are good for lows but can worsen the overall course of bipolar disorder by causing irritability, mood swings, and rapid cycling. To reduce this risk, bipolar patients receive either a mood stabilizer or an antipsychotic (or too often, both) in addition to the antidepressant. But striving to prevent harm from antidepressants comes at a potentially heavy cost. The side effects of the mood-stabilizing drugs are dangerous weight gain, diabetes, and heart disease. The tough question is how to draw the diagnostic line between bipolar and unipolar to balance the risks of taking versus the risks of not taking the mood-stabilizing medication.

The question is easy for patients having classic manic episodes who are clearly bipolar. Manic episodes are unmistakable and unforgettable. The person is supercharged in thought and deed; racing around; talking under pressure; spouting grandiose ideas, heightened creativity, a wild succession of totally impossible schemes; joking nonstop; floating on an elevated mood, but irritable if crossed; spending money like a drunken sailor; feeling boundless energy; acting inappropriately and impulsively; being intrusively sexual; and needing little sleep. Your Aunt Tillie could make the diagnosis of classic mania in a minute. And it provides a clear and essential call to action—no antidepressants without the safety net of a covering mood stabilizer.

But what do we do if the person doesn't have a full manic episode but does have periodic elevations in mood that are very different from his normal state? These less-than-full manic episodes are called "hypomanic" and they represent a conundrum. Patients who have alternating periods of depression and hypomania are at the crucial boundary separating bipolar and unipolar disorder. They could have been classified in either camp. If we classify them as bipolar, they will receive mood-stabilizing medication that may prevent rapid cycling, but they might be exposed to unnecessary mood-stabilizing medication that could be quite harmful. If we classify them as unipolar, they will receive only antidepressant medication, and this may trigger a manic episode. Faced with these ambiguous cards, we chose to add a new category, bipolar II, to describe patients who have depressions and hypomanic episodes. The weight of the evidence on their course, family history, and treatment response suggested they sorted better with bipolar disorder. And, on balance, we decided they could be more harmed receiving antidepressants without coverage than by the added burden of mood stabilizers. A close call, but it seemed safer to include bipolar II.

But there are vulnerabilities in the definition and assessment of bipolar II that gave the drug companies lots of wiggle room. There is no clear boundary between hypomania and simply feeling good—so advertisements began suggesting that even slight shifts upward in mood or passing irritability might be a subtle sign of bipolar disorder. This pitch could work especially well with depressed patients, who would have a lot of trouble distinguishing between being "high" and a return of normal mood. Street drugs or antidepressant medications can also provoke brief periods of elevated mood—should this be bipolar disorder?

We knew that bipolar II would expand the bipolar category somewhat into unipolar territory, but we did not think that it would double. Undoubtedly our decision resulted in more accurate diagnosis and safer treatment for many previously missed truly bipolar patients. But like all fads, it overshot and has led to unnecessary medication for many unipolar patients who have been misdiagnosed as bipolar on very flimsy grounds and are now receiving unnecessary mood stabilizing drugs.[25,26]

Why the big jump? It was the same old story of misleading drug company marketing. The bipolar market is potentially much larger than the schizophrenic market, so the drug companies pounced on bipolar II. The pitch in selling the ill was that any sign of irritability, agitation, temper, or elevated mood indicated a tendency to bipolar disease. Bipolar was everywhere in conferences and journals, on TV, in magazines, in the movies. Psychiatrists, primary care doctors, other mental health workers, patients, and families were bombarded with warnings on the perils of previously "missed" bipolar disorder.

Which brings up the question—knowing what we know now about the fad it caused, was it a good idea to add bipolar II to *DSM-IV*? I simply don't know. The pluses and minuses balance pretty closely. But one thing is clear—in boundary cases where the call is close, people shouldn't jump on the bipolar bandwagon created by drug company hype. The antipsychotic drugs are too risky to take unless there is a real reason.

Social Phobia Makes Shyness an Illness

Social phobia has turned everyday shyness into the third most common mental disorder, with rates ranging from 7 to a ridiculous 13 percent, depending on how loosely it is diagnosed. At least fifteen million adults would qualify for social phobia in the United States alone, making it a prime target for drug advertising. Shyness is a ubiquitous and perfectly normal human trait with the enormous survival value of keeping people safe rather than sorry. You want your tribe to have some exploratory types eager to venture out when the old water hole runs dry. And it is nice to have some aggressive types when the neighbors get feisty. But for your day-in, day-out survival under stable conditions, avoidance of the new and untried must have been the smart play. Otherwise, the DNA favoring avoidance wouldn't have survived to be so common.

Of course, there are some people whose social anxiety is totally incapacitating and enough to meet anyone's definition of mental disorder. But these are rare individuals, far too small a market ever to interest the drug company. Pharma's brilliance was to see past these few—to envision a world where even slightly excessive shyness could be magically transformed into a mental illness that would require a drug fix.

The statistical normality of shyness was exactly what gave the drug company a big fat marketing target. There is no clear boundary separating normal shyness from the mental disorder social anxiety. So the company began an all-out campaign to convince all shy people that they are sick and will miss out if they don't take the cure. It turns out conveniently that a number of public figures are really painfully shy and ready to shill ringing testimonials to the liberation that comes from owning up to the diagnosis and finally receiving proper treatment. Doctors were also blitzed and softened so as to be ready to prescribe Paxil when prospective "patients" followed the advertising command to "Ask your doctor." Before long, social anxiety disorder emerged from its lowly status as a rare psychiatric footnote and became a blossoming diagnostic star, one of the most common and commonly treated of the mental disorders.[27]

Social anxiety had a second feature that made it a marketing dream. Because most of the people who get the diagnosis are not really sick, it is easy to get them well. This is a population with an appallingly high placebo response rate. For the drug companies, this was actually appealingly high. Once someone (who wasn't really sick) got better due to the placebo effects of a drug (he never really needed), he was likely to stay on it as a good luck charm so as not to risk rocking the boat. He became a longtime loyal customer getting no benefit but set up for unnecessary complications.[28]

In preparing *DSM-IV*, we did not give social anxiety much attention. It didn't seem to be a diagnosis of great import to psychiatry. And until several years later, when it was blown up and abused by misleading advertising, it wasn't really of much interest. But we clearly had our collective heads in the sand and badly miscalculated. Our definition of social anxiety should have set an extremely high threshold to filter in only the really incapacitated and to filter out the merely uncomfortable. It is possible the smart advertising types could have overcome any definitional resistance on our part, but with greater foresight we could have put up a better fight.[29]

Major Depression Is Not Always So Major

Major depressive disorder (MDD) sometimes lives up to its ominous-sounding name; sometimes it doesn't. At its worst, MDD is one of mankind's cruelest afflictions. The emotional pain is worse than anything imaginable, worse than losing your closest love. But a lot of what passes for major depressive disorder is not really "major," is not really "depressive," and is not really "disorder." Loose diagnosis has created a false epidemic of MDD, with fifteen million Americans now qualifying at any given time. The transformation of expectable sadness into clinical depression has turned us into an overmedicated, pill-popping population.

The *DSM* definition of MDD is one of the most stable in the book, remaining essentially unchanged since its initial development in *DSM-III* in 1980—an endurance that reflects its usefulness. But there is a fatal flaw. Because the same criteria set defines both the most and the least severe depressions, it was written to meet the needs of both. The MDD definition works well at the severe end, but at the mild end it has led to the creeping repackaging of everyday normal unhappiness into mental disorder.

Mild major depression is a peculiar contradiction in terms; the descriptors "mild" and "major" are awkwardly juxtaposed and internally inconsistent. This semantic clumsiness reflects a clinical conundrum. There is no way to demarcate a clean boundary between the milder forms of clinical depression and severer forms of ordinary, normal sadness. If we try to diagnose everyone who really has major depression, inevitably we will misdiagnose many people who are simply having a rough patch in their lives that needs no medical label and requires no treatment.

There has been much controversy whether antidepressants work better than placebos precisely because many patients treated in studies are not very depressed or not depressed at all and really don't need an active medication.

Sadness should not be synonymous with sickness. There is no diagnosis for every disappointment or a pill for every problem. Life's difficulties—divorce, illness, job loss, financial troubles, interpersonal conflicts—can't be legislated away. And our natural reactions to them—sadness, dissatisfaction, and discouragement—shouldn't all be medicalized as mental disorder or treated with a pill. We are usually resilient, lick our wounds, mobilize our resources and our friends, and get on with it. Our capacity to feel emotional pain has great adaptive value equivalent in its purpose to physical pain—a signal that something has gone wrong. We can't convert all emotional pain into mental disorder without radically changing who we are, dulling the palette of our experience. If we can't tolerate sadness, we can't experience joy. Huxley's dystopian *Brave New World* shows how quickly pain-free translates into brain-dead.

The *DSMs* have made it too easy to get a diagnosis of MDD. The biggest weakness is not recognizing the role of severe life stress in causing reactive sadness. Suppose something terrible happens and you respond with two weeks of sadness, loss of interest and energy, and trouble sleeping and eating. Sounds perfectly understandable and completely normal, but *DSM* tags it major depressive disorder. The "epidemic" of MDD initiated by the loose *DSM* definitions was then driven by a combination of biological reductionism among physicians and fancy drug company marketing. Doctors bought the story line that all depression results from a chemical imbalance in the brain and therefore requires a chemical fix—the prescription of an antidepressant medication. This is absolutely true for severe depressions, absolutely false for most milder ones. The proof of this pudding is that psychotherapy is just as effective as medication for milder depressions, and neither has a big edge over placebo. Millions of people take medicine they don't need for a diagnosis of MDD that they don't really have, on the false assumption of chemical imbalance.[30,31,32]

I have saved the most sobering question for last. Suppose we had appropriately raised the thresholds for major depressive disorder so that it lived up to its name and no longer overinclusively captured the aches, pains, and sufferings of everyday life. Would this return to a saner and tighter diagnosis of MDD have resulted in saner prescription habits cutting into the excessive sales of Prozac, Zoloft, Paxil, Celexa, and the others? Or would 11 percent of the population still be taking antidepressants whether or not there is a clear diagnostic indication for them? How relevant was the excessive diagnosis of depression in supporting the vast overtreatment with antidepressants?

There is no way of knowing for sure. Certainly *DSM-IV* legitimizes the easy availability of antidepressants by fostering depressive diagnosis. But there is a recent historical precedent illustrating that promiscuous prescribing can occur even if there is no specific diagnosis to prescribe for. The antianxiety drugs Valium and Librium ruled the 1970s and 1980s with a dominance almost as impressive as that enjoyed now by antidepressants—and without a clear target diagnosis. It may be that the American public, under the auspices of profit-driven drug companies and careless doctors, will pop one pill or another whatever the *DSM* chooses to say or not say.

There is another historical precedent—a much older one going back all the way to shaman times. The wisdom of the ages is that whenever they feel bad, people want to take something to feel better. The five-thousand-year-old mummified man, wonderfully preserved in the ice of the Alps, was carrying his little bag of plant medicine—the Prozac of his day. As we have seen, most medicine taken for most illnesses, most of the time, since the dawn of time, has at best been of very little specific help, usually has been completely inert, and very often has been directly harmful, even poisonous. But shamans, priests, and doctors prescribed them and patients dutifully took them and seemed to benefit. The magic of medication manages to survive its ineffectuality and potential harm. The popularity of placebo seems to be built into our DNA.

My medical purism rebels against the idea that millions of people are taking expensive, potentially harmful, largely placebo medication for a psychiatrically endorsed, drug company promoted "illness" that is really no more than an expectable discomfort or existential problem, inevitable in life as we know it. For a significant percentage of people with mild or transient symptoms, SSRIs are nothing more than very expensive, potentially harmful placebos. There are better ways to deal with sadness. People should have more faith in the remarkable healing powers of time, natural resilience, exercise, family and social support, and psychotherapy—and much less automatic faith in chemical imbalance and pills. There is some good news from *DSM-5* on this issue. Under much external pressure, *DSM-5* makes it easier to withhold the diagnosis of MDD when the person's sadness is an understandable reaction to loss or stress.

Of course, none of this applies when the depression is persistent or more severe. It is a shame and a tragedy that one third of the people with severe and incapacitating MDD get no treatment whatever for it. Medications would be enormously valuable in these situations when they are so sorely needed, but instead they have been oversold for situations when they are not. I would prefer a psychiatry doing what it can do well, taking care of the really sick who need and can benefit from our help—not wasting time, money, and effort turning normal into mental disorder.

Post-Traumatic Stress Disorder: Hard to Get Right

Of all the many conditions in *DSM-IV*, post-traumatic stress disorder (PTSD) is paradoxically one of the most underdiagnosed and also one of the most overdiagnosed. Errors in both directions are common and easy to make; I know this well because I have made them both ways. PTSD is missed when people suffer its symptoms stoically and in silence. PTSD is overdiagnosed when it is a trigger for financial gain.

PTSD has probably been with us since the birth of humanity. Our ancestors were slow, weak creatures exposed and dreadfully vulnerable at the water hole. Life was always at risk, likely to be "nasty, brutish, and short." Death lurked everywhere—unpredictable, sudden, and often violent. The human reaction to trauma is a great equalizer—regardless of all the differences in our personalities or previous life experiences, we all have the same set of remarkably uniform and stereotypical symptoms in response to a life-threatening stress. We relive the moment over and over and over again in a profoundly emotional way. Images, memories, or flashbacks bring it alive again, intruding incessantly during the day, and at night there are terrifying dreams. Anything resembling the event cues avoidance and terror. Every strange male face is a reminder of the rapist. A car backfiring is a reminder of being under rifle fire. Driving seems impossibly difficult after a bad car accident because the driver keeps visualizing the accident about to happen again. This set of reactions must have had enormous survival value—providing an absolutely indelible object lesson in the importance of avoiding similar dangers in the future. It was the ultimate in powerful one-trial learning—our ancestors had to learn fast and learn well because predators don't often give second chances.

Almost everyone has at least some intrusive imagery and emotional reactivity to cues after a shocking event—this is part of the human condition and until recently was not defined as illness. For most people the intrusive images gradually become less intrusive and the triggers become less terrifying. The mental disorder PTSD should be diagnosed only when the symptoms persist and cause significant disability. At the severe extreme, PTSD can become chronic and incapacitating. Life is filled with haunting memories and scary triggers. It feels empty, stale, flat, and without meaning. The suicide rate is high.

What determines whether the reaction is transient enough to be considered normal versus devastating enough to be a mental disorder? A lot has to do with the nature and duration of the trauma. PTSD is more likely the more terrible the stress, the longer it lasts, the more intense and intimate the exposure, the more helpless the person feels. Someone who is shot is more at risk than someone who sees the shooting, and seeing is more risky that just hearing the shot at a distance. Horrors intentionally inflicted by humans—torture, rape, and assault—tend to cause worse symptoms than accidents or natural catastrophes. The course also depends on the person and his context. People who have had more emotional troubles before the trauma are more likely to have worse and more prolonged reactions to it. And traumas accumulate—the more one experiences, the greater the risk of PTSD. Family, job, support systems, and treatment are healing; drinking or using substances makes things much worse.

Although PTSD is straightforward and absolutely characteristic on paper, its accurate evaluation in real life is often difficult or impossible. The first part of the definition—describing the nature of the traumatic stress—is easy. It has to be absolutely terrifying, far beyond the expectable problems that plague our everyday life. Rape, assault, totaling a car, natural disaster, torture, war, violent death or injury of a loved one—these all qualify. Nonviolent disasters—divorce, job loss, financial catastrophe, romantic disappointment—these don't cause PTSD.

But then things get difficult. The diagnosis of PTSD is imprecise because it is based exclusively on the person's own self-report—there is no laboratory test or objective measure. It is inherently difficult for people to accurately report their reactions to an overwhelmingly terrible event. Many and complex psychological and contextual factors may lead them, consciously or unconsciously, to downplay or to exaggerate symptoms. It is no surprise that rates of PTSD in returning veterans can vary so dramatically—just a few percent to as high as 20 percent—depending on how the diagnosis is made and which country is surveyed, even if the troops have had similar wartime experiences.[33]

Underreporting helps people reduce fear and pain in the short run, but at great cost in the long. It is in the very nature of PTSD that people suffering from it will attempt to avoid reminders. Who wants to keep describing and reliving the worst moment in his life? Some will fear that talking about symptoms will make them worse or cause a breakdown. Some are too depressed to speak of the pain. And some under-reporting is macho, particularly among military types who prefer to brave out debilitating symptoms rather than admit to what they regard as weakness in having them.

Overdiagnosis is also easy. Everyone has some PTSD symptoms after going through something horrible, but these usually wear off without causing long-term or clinically significant hardship. Symptoms are more likely to persist and be interpreted in their worst light if significant financial gain is attached to having them. All other emotional problems, both preexisting and subsequent, may be incorporated into the PTSD experience. Patienthood can become a way of life and rationale for people who are struggling for other reasons. On the military side, PTSD is incentivized because the diagnosis qualifies someone for otherwise unavailable disability and health benefits. In civilian life, the most frequent context for overdiagnosis is the assignment of workmen's compensation or of damage awards in legal suits. The overdiagnosis is not necessarily a question of conscious manipulation (although faking certainly does happen); symptoms just tend to take on more consequence when money is at stake.[34]

PTSD is one fad that has not been much instigated by drug companies. They shy away from advertising for it because medicines are not very effective and they fear the risk of bad publicity when things don't go well in patients with such high visibility.

The Sexual Revolution

Sex has always been sexy to the world at large but something of a bore to psychiatry. The field boasts only a small handful of experts, attracts almost no research funding, has a thin professional literature, and is a very small part of most clinical practice. I had more than the usual exposure as part of my job as head of the outpatient clinic at the Cornell University/New York Hospital during the 1980s and 1990s. One of the stars of our faculty was Helen Singer Kaplan, a glamorous pioneer in the field. Why pioneer? It was she who popularized the notion that the sexual disorders should reflect problems occurring in each of the stages of the sexual act: desire, arousal, and orgasm. Helen was the person most responsible for shaping the *DSM-III* sexual disorders, and her influence is enduring because this section has remained stable through subsequent *DSMs*.[35]

Why glamorous? Helen had personal style, but beyond that she had a practical hands-on attitude to sex therapy that seemed shockingly direct but was probably very effective. In her private practice, she made use of a stable of "sexual surrogates"—breathtakingly beautiful, sexually wise assistant therapists who taught the ropes to Helen's male patients and were perfectly capable of rekindling anyone's flagging desire. Helen claimed her surrogates got incredible results—and I certainly believe they could work wonders. Another of Helen's sidekicks—Dr. Ruth Westheimer—had a completely different claim to fame and an improbable TV and radio stardom. "Dr. Ruth" got great ratings by being the tiny old grandmother who could cheerfully rattle off the graphic details of the most intimate sexual acts, in a delightful Old World accent.

For *DSM-IV*, the sexual disorders represented the stillest backwater of psychiatry, our least important task. We had a sexual disorders work group that sifted through the limited literature, offered very few suggestions, did no field trials. It was a relief to have at least one section of the manual that required so little work.

This was the quiet before an unanticipated storm. Several years after *DSM-IV* was published, the sexual disorders exploded off its dull pages to become the marketing hit of a lifetime. Viagra changed the world, becoming one of the best-selling drugs in history and turning an obscure sexual disorder into a ubiquitous lifestyle issue. Viagra could not have risen to its heights of fame and fortune without first convincing the world that "erectile dysfunction" (affectionately nick-named ED for the TV and print ads) was a ubiquitous problem that could occur even in the seemingly hardy.

The first step was to persuade old folks to come out of the closet and own up to their ED. A brilliantly designed ad campaign managed to purchase the services of the world's most perfect shill. Bob Dole, on the rebound from losing to the much younger (and obviously more virile) Bill Clinton in the 1996 presidential election, started a second and more lucrative career as the poster boy of Viagra and the champion of rejuve-nated geriatric sex. The implication was that Viagra provided a fountain of youth that could expand virility and vitality even for guys too old to be president. And if someone as famous as good old Bob could man up on TV and admit to having ED, why not bring up your problem in the privacy of your doctor's consulting room? The message—you owe it to yourself and to the little lady to be all you can possibly be. With Viagra on board, seventy was to become the new forty.

But why stop with the geriatric set, and its necessarily narrow market, when there is so much product to sell, so little time. Soon no one of any age could possibly hide from the long reach of ED; no bed-room was safe from its chilling grip. ED was everywhere, featured on all media all the time.

The marketing of ED required that its threshold be pushed ever lower. ED started as a medical condition applying only to a small population of sufferers with well-established flaccidity. Soon Viagra became a general potency tonic. If it could raise the dead, just imagine what a grand slam home run it could hit for the living. Sex pills went from being a medical treatment to a performance enhancer and an insurance policy protecting against that occasional off day. After all, a wise man is always armed and loaded to the hilt. ED had outgrown the narrow confines of psychiatry and medicine. It was more than just another "epidemic"; it was a lifestyle choice worthy of consideration by every couple. Viagra to the rescue to make the man of the house truly a man in full. The selling of ED was a total success.

Well, almost total. So far the sexual dysfunction story had pretty much left out half the human race, not something that sits well with the drug company financial types or their marketing geniuses. Women had surely made their lovely appearance in some of the Viagra ads, exuding the unbelievable satisfaction that comes from consorting with a Viagra man. But she was decidedly the sidekick and trophy, not the primary target of the campaign. This was unacceptable to the dignity (and greed) of the Pharma machine. Certainly women have sexual dysfunctions too. They are described right there in black-and-white in *DSM-IV*. If they have the ill, let's set about the job of selling them the pill.

There was one small problem—no real evidence that Viagra works for women. The other products being hawked (e.g., testosterone patches) were also not all that effective and had problematic side effects. But no matter, let's create the disorder and the customers will come. This marketing tale is well spelled out by Ray Moynihan in his well-researched book with the wonderful title *Sex, Lies, and Pharmaceuticals*. The ploy was to redefine expectable glitches in normal female sexuality into an almost ubiquitous "female sexual dysfunction" (FSD).[36]

The best hook for selling FSD was the use (really, misuse) of surveys asking women about their sexual experience. It became widely reported, and accepted as established fact, that 43 percent of women had FSD. These results were remarkable—a marketing godsend and triumph. Previously obscure *DSM* sexual disorders were being inflated into something that actually transcended mere epidemic. The expectable sexual experience of almost one half of women had been repackaged as FSD.

One symptom does not a diagnosis make. Asking a woman seven questions about her sex life and concluding she has an illness if she responds positively to any one of them is either naive or intellectually dishonest. It leaves out altogether the determination of whether there is a necessary cluster of symptoms and whether these cause enough distress to warrant clinical attention. Women who checked a box were often not troubled by having a less than completely perfect sex life; nor did they usually see themselves as having a medical problem. Not every woman wanted or expected to live a *Sex and the City* lifestyle.

The sexual revolution in drug marketing is the most blatant widening of a narrow medical indication into a performance-enhancing, cosmetic, lifestyle "treatment." It is also the most evident exhibition of the raw power and profitability of advertising to sell attitudes, illness, and product. *DSM-IV* was no match for all this muscle, easily misused or sidestepped. Also lost in the pill-pushing shuffle were sexual and relational psychotherapies that might bring lasting benefit, not just real or imagined symptomatic improvement.

Rape Is a Crime, Not a Mental Disorder

This a cautionary tale of legal loopholes, Supreme Court dithering, and *DSM-IV* foul-ups—all combining to create constitutional violations and a terrible misuse of psychiatry.

The story begins with a laudable legal reform that had unanticipated dreadful consequences. Thirty years ago, the civil rights movement became rightly concerned that blacks were getting longer prison terms than whites for committing equivalent crimes. The answer was to substitute fixed sentencing for each type of crime instead of allowing the previously indeterminate (and possibly biased) judicial discretion. This was meant to guarantee uniformity, predictability, and fairness. To keep the total number of prison beds constant (and thus not raise costs), the fixed sentence for each crime was set at the average of what had before been a wide range. For rape, this was seven years. A brutal serial rapist (who previously might have pulled twenty-five years from a disapproving judge) now was limited to a term of only seven. The result was predictable, but not predicted. Brutal recidivists used their premature freedom to rape again, often soon after release from prison and in the most despicable ways possible.

The ensuing public outrage inspired a legal loophole to keep rapists locked up. Twenty states and the federal government passed "sexually violent predator" (SVP) laws that allowed the continued psychiatric incarceration of offenders if it could be shown that they had a mental disorder. At the end of their prison terms, the prisoner would become a mental patient, transferred involuntarily to a psychiatric "hospital" that actually quite closely resembled a prison. Few of the railroaded SVPs ever accepted a "treatment" format that allowed whatever they said to be used against them in later hearings. Even among those who complete the "treatment," few ever achieve release.

From the public safety standpoint, this lifetime-within-walls approach was a brilliant solution, a convenient way to keep possibly dangerous rapists from prowling the streets. But there is a downside that presents a different set of dangers—the statutes strike straight to the heart of hard-won constitutional protections against preventive detention and double jeopardy. The wise legal saying is that "bad cases make for bad law." Thousands of undesirable rapists have been confined for the best of motives, but using the worst of methods and creating a slippery slope erosion of precious constitutional protections.

Which brings us to Supreme Court dithering. In three close and remarkably ambiguous rulings, the Court supported the constitutionality of this convenient parking of SVPs—but emphasized that it is legal only when the rapist has a mental disorder that made him do it. The U.S. Constitution doesn't allow preventive detention for criminals no matter how dangerous they are feared to be, but it does allow long-term involuntary treatment for mental patients. The Supreme Court approval of SVP commitment depends completely on the presumed ability to distinguish individuals whose sexual dangerousness arises from sickness rather than common criminality. Lacking the presence of mental disorder, enforced incarceration in a psychiatric hospital-cum-prison would clearly represent a deprivation of due process and a violation of civil rights. Our Constitution does not allow us to turn all about-to-be-released prisoners into unwilling patients, just because we fear they may possibly still be dangerous.

The constitutionality of the SVP statutes rests on having a meaningful way of distinguishing the mentally ill sex offender from the simple criminal. Given three chances, the Supreme Court refused to provide guidelines on the critical question of what constitutes a qualifying diagnosis. Unfortunately, the state statutes are also far too vague to be of any help. The American Psychiatric Association does have an unequivocal position. Rape as a mental disorder was considered in the last four *DSM* revisions (*DSM-III*, *DSM-IIIR*, *DSM-IV*, and *DSM-5*) and definitively rejected by all of them and also by a special task force report. Rape is a crime, not a mental disorder.[37]

But what was the legal system to do with potentially dangerous rapists awaiting their release dates? This is where a *DSM-IV* foul-up played its part. The very worst writing in all of *DSM-IV* is concentrated in the sexual disorders section. Not anticipating the later misuse of *DSM-IV* in SVP hearings, our wording was imprecise and did not provide adequate protection against the stretching of the definition of mental disorder to include rape. Zealous, misinformed, and highly paid evaluators, employed by the government, badly misinterpreted the intent of *DSM-IV* and began the strange practice of diagnosing the act of rape as itself an indication of the presence of a qualifying mental disorder that would justify psychiatric incarceration. The evaluators ignored the many forms of criminal intent that motivate rape—callously grabbing opportunity, drug disinhibition, poor impulse control, exerting power, revenge, profiting from the sex trade, gangbanger peer pressure, wartime mayhem, and so on. Instead, rape was magically medicalized, in the service of legal and public safety expediency, to allow preventive detention and deprive rapists of their civil rights.

Regarding rape as a mental disorder violates common sense and time-honored legal precedent. Rape has always been treated as a crime, never as a sickness. The Bible says so; the much older Code of Hammurabi says so, and, in fact, so does every legal code ever written. Punishments have varied. In tribal law, the female victim is treated as private property that has lost some of its value after the rape. The rapist therefore has to pay off her father, husband, or other owner. Later systems, with more respect for women, treat rape not just as a matter of lost financial value, but rather as a crime against the women and the state. Never before has rape ever received legal recognition as a sickness and never before has the incarceration of rapists been psychiatric, rather than penal.

Rapists are always bad people, very rarely mad people. They should not be able to use mental disorder as a legal excuse, but neither should rape be a legal excuse for mental hospitalization. Rapists should be kept off the streets with very long prison sentences, not loopholed into involuntary psychiatric commitment. Once they have served their time, they should be released, as would any other common criminal.

My concern does not arise from any sympathy for rapists. Instead my fear is that treating them unfairly greases that slippery slope to a more general degradation of the Constitution, lessening respect for the sacred values of due process and the protection of civil liberties. The frightening experience of other countries should counsel caution in ours. Psychiatry has elsewhere been dangerously abused by the penal system to stifle political dissent, economic complaints, or individual difference. A legal system willing to compromise its constitutional principles to deal with inconvenient rapists may in the future stretch further to use psychiatry against those with inconvenient political goals, religious beliefs, or sexual preferences.[38]

As Robert Musil pointed out seventy years ago, "The angel of medicine, if he has listened too long to lawyer's arguments, too often forgets his own mission. He then folds his wings with a clatter and conducts himself in court like a reserve angel of the court."[39]

The Lesson

Even if you do most things pretty much right in preparing a diagnostic manual (and we didn't do a bad job with *DSM-IV*), you don't get to control how it will be used and misused once it is published and the genie is out of the bottle. We must take partial responsibility for the epidemics of autism, attention deficit, and adult bipolar disorder. But epidemics are driven by many other powerful and converging forces: the drug company's aggressive selling of diagnoses; reckless thought leaders; gullible patients and doctors; advocacy groups; the media; the Internet; and social networking. Some inflating influences are diagnosis specific: school systems encouraging the diagnosis of autism or ADD as a qualification for extra services or the VA requiring a PTSD diagnosis for health and disability benefits. Others are general trends—the unrealistic expectation of so many people in our society that they, and their children, not only be perfect but also feel perfect.

DSM-IV was a bit player in the continuing march of diagnostic inflation. The major engine was drug company marketing. Three years after *DSM-IV* was published, Pharma lobbyists finagled an unprecedented reversal in federal regulations to allow advertising directly to consumers. This was the key to the kingdom. In the next decade, the companies tripled spending on marketing—selling depression, ADHD, bipolar, social phobia, and sexual disorders with the same enthusiasm that Coca-Cola sells pop. The ads were usually misleading but devastatingly effective. Patients self-misdiagnosed and asked their doctor for the magic pill that would correct their chemical imbalance. The doctors listened. Patients who requested a drug they had seen advertised were seventeen times more likely to walk out of the office with a prescription. The massive advertising had put the companies in charge of diagnosis. In the excitement, I doubt that many people were checking the fine print of *DSM-IV* criteria sets to ensure that there was a good fit. *DSM-IV* had lost control of the system—assuming we ever had it. There are no defenders of normality, nothing to prevent the constant creep of diagnosis. It is an unfair fight. Humpty Dumpty was certainly not calling the shots.

DSM-IV didn't by itself do much harm, but we certainly didn't do much good (unless you give us dubious credit for not making a bad situation worse). On paper, we won most of the battles to contain diagnostic spread—but we badly lost the war to the outside forces that determined how *DSM-IV* would be used. I really don't know whether a more aggressively revised and deflating *DSM-IV*, with markedly raised thresholds, would have been feasible or effective. However, in retrospect, knowing what I know now, I regret that we didn't do the experiment. We probably could not have stopped diagnostic inflation, but I would feel better if we had gone down fighting, rather than just standing pat with what turned out to be a losing hand.

CHAPTER 6

Fads of the Future

Pride goeth before the fall.
PROVERBS 16:18

DSM-5 HAS JUST been published—not a happy moment in the history of psychiatry or for me personally. It risks turning diagnostic inflation into hyperinflation—further cheapening the currency of psychiatric diagnosis and unleashing a wave of new false epidemics.[1,2] The economic equivalent would be printing up loads of new money when prices are already rising way too fast. *DSM-5* is a cautionary tale of soaring ambition, poor execution, and a closed process. The good news is that a last-minute reform effort, instigated by a new leadership team at the American Psychiatric Association, eliminated about one third of the worst changes that would have opened the floodgates of diagnostic inflation even further. The bad news is that, despite this, *DSM-5* kept the other two thirds and will significantly add to, not correct, the already existing problems of overdiagnosis and overtreatment.[3]

Ambition—Icarus Flies Too High and Flames Out

In preparing any *DSM*, it is wise to be extremely modest—underpromise and then work like hell to overperform. *DSM-5* got this backward—it wildly overpromised, then failed to meet minimal performance standards.

The excessive *DSM-5* ambition to effect a paradigm shift in psychiatric diagnosis expressed itself in three different initiatives. First was the unrealistic goal of transforming psychiatric diagnosis by somehow basing it on the exciting findings of neuroscience. This would be wonderful were it possible, but the effort failed for the obvious reason that it is still a bridge too far. Neuroscience will inform everyday psychiatric diagnosis only at its own slow and steady pace; it cannot be rushed forward before its time—and that time is decidedly not yet.

Ambitious goal two was to expand the boundary of clinical psychiatry—copying other specialties of medicine by pursuing the brave new world of early illness identification and preventive treatment. The irony, of course, is that excessive early screening is just now being discredited across many of the medical specialties that had served as the exemplars for *DSM-5*.

The third *DSM-5* ambition is the least dangerous and most attainable. The idea is to make psychiatric diagnosis more precise by quantifying disorders with numbers, rather than merely naming them. Done well, this would be a good idea—but *DSM-5* developed unnecessarily complex dimensional ratings that could never be used clinically.[4,5]

Icarus flew too close to the sun, melted his wings, and fell into the sea. *DSM-5* tried to achieve three impossibly ambitious paradigm shifts in psychiatry and failed in all three. The messy process undeservedly tarred the credibility of psychiatry—the field is a lot better than anyone would assume watching the *DSM-5* follies unfold. Trying to be great prevented *DSM-5* from being good enough.[6]

Methods Matter

DSM-5 was not prepared with method in mind. Distracted by fantasies of creativity, it ignored mundane necessities like efficiency, punctuality, consistency, and quality control. Doing a *DSM* is not conceptually difficult. The tough part is attending to all the organizational details. It requires constant monitoring of the work groups to ensure they are following the common goal and preparing a consistent product. The organizational principle that brought cohesion to *DSM-III* and *DSM-IIIR* was the omnipresent leadership of Bob Spitzer, who chaired every work group, nursed every detail, and wrote every word. For *DSM-IV*, the glue was a set of standard operating procedures. Every methodological issue was spelled out in detail well before the work began. There were explicit criteria for making changes and a centralized method for the literature review, data reanalyses, and field trials. In contrast, *DSM-5* was a hodgepodge of disorganized method. Work groups were instructed to be innovative but were provided no clear marching orders that would cohere their separate productions. Not surprisingly, the different groups varied widely in the methods, thoroughness, quality, impartiality, and clarity of their reviews. Perhaps most puzzling was the inability of the *DSM-5* to plan ahead or meet its own deadlines. The original publication date had to be pushed back two years. Even with this added time there was a mad scramble at the end—and *DSM-5* had to cancel its crucial quality control step when work fell so far behind there was no time left to complete it.

There is a much better way. Evidence-based medicine has made enormous strides in specifying how research findings should be translated into clinical practice. The *DSM-5* literature reviews should have been conducted by independent evaluators who would have had the dual advantages of special expertise in evidence-based methods and impartiality, with no pet proposals to protect. Work group members are experts on their diagnoses, but not experts in thorough and impartial literature review and risk/benefit analysis. There is also no possible excuse for all the missed deadlines and for canceling much needed quality control.

To Change or Not to Change

Psychiatry's research revolution is exciting only on the basic science side (elucidating brain function); we are undeniably in a deep rut when it comes to progress in clinical diagnosis and treatment. There has been no real advance in diagnosis since *DSM-III* in 1980, and no real advance in treatment since the early 1990s. Psychiatric diagnosis doesn't need much updating, much less a paradigm shift. Given a steady state, a pragmatist will move carefully and only in small steps. If something new comes along that brings obvious value at low risk, grab it—but don't change just for the sake of being different.[7]

Playing with the diagnostic system can lead to all sorts of unintended consequences. If we can't be confident about the impact of something new, it is better not to change the old. Even if you check things out as carefully as you can, the future is impossible to predict. The only safe bet is that if something can possibly go wrong, it probably will. Recent *DSM* history teaches us that whatever changes are made will be subject to unexpected misinterpretation and misuse under pressure from drug companies, school services, disability requirements, and the legal system. If there is any possible loophole with an incentive for gain, someone will drive a truck through it. Having withstood time's test, the old tried and true should be changed only for very good cause.[8]

Aside from risk, changes come at considerable cost. Most expensive is the broken continuity between the findings of past and future research. How can one interpret differences in results of studies of the same diagnosis done before versus after the change? Arbitrary changes are also upsetting to clinicians, patients, teachers, students, and administrators. Everything would seem to favor a look-before-you-leap prudence. The *DSM-5* leadership initially took just the opposite tack—valuing change seemingly for the sake of change accompanied by lack of interest in understanding why things were as they were. The rhetoric supporting this radical position was the need to have the diagnostic system reflect rapid advances in science—a misleading conflation of the growth spurt in basic science with the dead stall in clinical science.[9]

Field Tests That Fail the Test

The *DSM-IV* trials were funded by the National Institute of Mental Heath after an extensive external peer review of their scientific method and merit. This was the most meticulously designed and carefully performed trial ever done. And yet we missed predicting the epidemics in ADHD, autism, and bipolar disorder. APA failed to attract external research funding for the *DSM-5* field trials and had to put up more than $3 million of its own money. The design of the study was created behind closed doors and never subjected to the much-needed peer review that might have corrected its obvious flaws. As a result, the *DSM-5* field trials tested the wrong question, in the wrong way, in the wrong settings, and with an unrealistic deadline. The results are impossible to interpret—a waste of time, money, effort, and talent.

DSM-5 asked the wrong question, focusing itself exclusively on the reliability of its new diagnostic proposals (whether psychiatrists can agree) and completely avoiding the much more important questions of practical utility: Will a new diagnosis help patients or harm them? For this, you need data on rates, accuracy, efficacy, and safety. And you need to get beyond readily available, but unrepresentative, samples provided by university hospitals and instead study how the criteria will work in real-life settings. For reasons I will never understand, *DSM-5* avoided asking the questions that really mattered.

Then it got worse. The design of the field trial was impossibly cumbersome to perform and lent itself to administrative confusion and sloppy implementation. It was obvious on first reading that the timeline was absurdly truncated—the trial would take at least twice as long as allocated. When finally the field trial limped to its much belated completion, the results it produced were an embarrassment. The reliability of the diagnoses tested in the *DSM-5* field trial were far below what had been achieved in the past and what could be achieved in the present if the project had been conducted competently. The taint of poor reliability stained even old standbys like major depressive disorder that had stood up to hundreds of previous tests conducted over forty years.

The original plan had included a quality control step. If diagnoses had poor reliability in Stage 1 (as many did), Stage 2 (rewriting and retesting) would correct them. But Stage 1 came in so late, there was no time left for Stage 2—if the 2013 publication date were to be met as required to meet APA budget projections for publishing profits. This was the moment of truth for *DSM-5*—a compelling test of its integrity.[10,11]

APA flunked—instead of admitting that its reliability results were unacceptable and seeking the necessary corrections that might meet historical standards, the goalposts were moved. Declaring by fiat that previous expectations were too high, *DSM-5* announced it would accept agreements among raters that were sometimes barely better than two monkeys throwing darts at a diagnostic board. The essential Stage 2 step of quality control was surreptitiously canceled and a premature *DSM-5* was rushed quickly to the printers to get sales moving and the cash register ringing. For me, this was perhaps the most dispiriting decision in the whole disappointing history of *DSM-5*. APA was not only sacrificing its own credibility but also putting patient safety at risk and unfairly tainting the whole mental health enterprise.

Follow the Money: Profits and Losses

APA has spent an astounding $25 million on *DSM-5*. I can't imagine where all that money went. *DSM-IV* cost only about $5 million, more than half of which came from outside research grants. Even if the *DSM-5* product were made of gold instead of lead, $25 million would be wildly out of proportion. The rampant disorganization of *DSM-5* must have caused colossal waste.

APA can't afford this kind of excess. It is in deficit, has reserves below what are recommended for a nonprofit, is rapidly losing members, has fewer people attending its annual meeting, and can no longer rely on questionable subsidies from the drug industry. The *DSM* publishing cash cow was its last hope to save the budget—forcing a publication schedule that couldn't be met with a quality product.

All along, APA has treated *DSM-5* more as private publishing asset than as public trust. First there were confidentiality agreements to protect "intellectual property," then an inappropriately aggressive protection of trademark and copyright, and finally the unseemly rush to prematurely publish because this was necessary to fill a budgetary hole. APA has an impossible conflict of interest in its dual role as fiduciary of the diagnostic system (a public trust) and beneficiary of publishing profits. Guild interest should never trump public interest—but it has.

Fads of the Future

DSM-5 has included several sure fire fads of the future. All have symptoms that are part of everyday life and commonly encountered in the general population. None has a definition precise enough to prevent the mislabeling of many people now considered normal. None has a treatment proven to be effective. All will likely lead to much unnecessary, and sometimes harmful, treatment or testing. The aggregate effects will be overdiagnosis, unnecessary stigma, overtreatment, a misallocation of resources,[12] and a negative impact in the way we see ourselves as individuals and as a society.[13]

Turning Tantrums into Psychiatric Disorder

Child psychiatrists often dare to go where no one has gone before—and children wind up paying the price. They keep inventing new ways to wildly overdiagnose psychiatric illness in kids. Previously I mentioned a study that found 83 percent of kids qualify for mental disorder diagnosis by the time they are twenty-one. Now the child researchers have taken it a step further—introducing a new *DSM-5* diagnosis that may get the number even closer to 100 percent. First called "temper dysregulation," then rechristened with the tongue-twisting disruptive mood dysregulation disorder (DMDD); the idea of turning temper tantrums into a mental disorder is terrible, however named. We should not have the ambition to label as mental disorder every inconvenient or distressing aspect of childhood.

The experts working on *DSM-5* meant well. Recognizing the catastrophic misdiagnosis of childhood bipolar disorder, they hoped to replace it with DMDD, which doesn't carry the same implication of lifetime illness and is less likely to be overmedicated with obesity-inducing drugs. This was a silly solution just on the face of it. The child experts were missing an obvious risk. Instead of simply replacing childhood bipolar, DMDD will likely become wildly overinclusive, used to describe all manner of kids who require no diagnosis at all or a more specific one. Kids have only so many ways of responding to the world and frequently resort to temper tantrums as a way of communicating anger and distress. Almost always, this is not indicative of a mental disorder but rather represents a developmental stage or a temperamental variant or a response to stress or a symptom of any number of mental disorders. "Run-of-the-mill" temper tantrums are usually best ignored; severe and persistent tantrums may require evaluation to determine their underlying cause; but temper tantrums by themselves should never be given the status of a separate official diagnosis. By turning a common, nonspecific symptom into a mental disorder, DMDD is likely to increase inappropriate antipsychotic use, not reduce it.

The research evidence on DMDD is almost nonexistent, based only on a few years of work by just one research group.[14] Nothing is known about its likely prevalence in the general population of kids; whether it can be distinguished from normal temper tantrums; its relation to all the many other disorders that present with angry outbursts; its course; its preferred treatment; and the trade-off between treatment response and adverse complications.

The criteria for diagnosing DMDD were pretty much conjured out of thin air and are not nearly restrictive enough. While trying to rescue kids currently misdiagnosed as bipolar, it will undoubtedly open the door to the misdiagnosis of normal kids who are going through a stage or are normally temperamental. There is no bright line distinguishing normal temper tantrums from abnormal ones. And there is enormous variability in what is considered appropriate across different families, subcultures, and developmental periods. Tantrums are so common precisely because they have had great survival value—natural selection favors the squeaky wheel, providing it with extra grease. Baby chimps dominate their parents just the same way.

The way the diagnosis of DMDD is made will vary greatly, depending on the tolerance of the clinician, family, school, and peer group. The "stresses" that trigger the episodes may be minimal in some cases but remarkably provocative and causing readily understandable temper outbursts in others. Family fights may be translated into individual psychopathology. In the heat of battle, it will doubtless be forgotten that most kids will outgrow their developmental or situational temper problems and gradually acquire self-control and better ways of getting needs met. My experience tells me that this unstudied diagnosis may well become very popular and will spread to normal kids, who would do a lot better without it.

Atypical antipsychotic drugs may be helpful in reducing some forms of explosive temper outbursts. But their beneficial effects for the few must be balanced against their very great dangers when used inappropriately for the many. Even in severely disturbed kids, there are serious clinical and ethical questions, but medicine may be needed in extremely exigent circumstances. In kids who have disturbing (but essentially "normal") developmental or situational storms or are irritable for other reasons (e.g., substance use, ADHD), antipsychotics are a disastrously bad choice. DMDD could turn out to be the most dangerous epidemic caused by *DSM-5*.[15] The sensible thing would have been to face down childhood bipolar directly with a bold warning against it in *DSM-5* and by carrying out a campaign to reeducate physicians, parents, and teachers previously brainwashed by pharmaceutical hype. Fighting fire with fire sometimes leads to more fire.

The Forgetting of Normal Aging Becomes a Disease

My wife, Donna, and I joke that we are in a race to the bottom to see who will become demented first; the loser gets to be caretaker. Trouble is, the joke is not all that funny and is getting less so as we both approach the finish line. We constantly forget where we have put keys, wallets, glasses, mail, books, papers, computers, BlackBerrys, clothing, phone numbers—you name it—and usually we blame each other for playful or malicious misplacing. We forget appointments, birthdays, movies seen last night, news just read, where the car is parked, or other recent events in our lives. I get lost frequently in the larger world; she is sometimes befuddled a few blocks from home. We are both terrible at remembering people's names, but at least Donna can still do faces.

Sounds pretty bad, and I guess it is. There are a few consolations. Donna manages to pay the bills, do the taxes, book the trips, organize the household, edit this book, and be the best-informed and smartest person I know. I can still write blogs and books, give talks, and give you the scoop on the Peloponnesian War. Most comforting, the people we know in our age group all have very similar tales of woe. None of us can see as well, hear as clearly, chew as efficiently, sleep as soundly, run as fast, do as many push-ups, climb as many flights, or hold as much water as our younger and stronger selves. This physical decrement with age doesn't get defined as sickness because it is expectable and inevitable.

In contrast, losing a mental step is now the *DSM-5* psychiatric illness mild neurocognitive disorder (MND). This diagnosis is intended to cover people who don't yet have dementia but who do have signs of mental decline that may put them at risk for later developing it. I would heartily endorse MND if there were a treatment for it or if it provided a really good way of predicting the future. But there is no treatment and little predictive power. If I gave myself this diagnosis, I wouldn't know what to do with it. Accepting mental aging makes more sense than diagnosing it until we have an accurate biological test or an effective treatment. Donna and I would not yet meet the criteria proposed for MND, but my guess is that the fine points of its criteria set will be ignored in general practice, and the diagnosis will be applied very loosely. MND will not be specific to those experiencing early symptoms of dementia but will soon broaden inappropriately to medicalize the gradual mental decline that is characteristic of normal aging.

This is not the intent of the sponsors. Their goal is to identify those at risk for Alzheimer's before they develop the full picture of dementia—with the hope that early diagnosis will lead eventually to early intervention, before the damage is done. Alzheimer's probably takes decades to evolve. The experts are excited by the prospect of becoming preventively proactive. Eventually, they hope that amyloid may be an early marker of Alzheimer's, in analogy to cholesterol with heart disease. Early identification and early treatment might prevent the worst ravages of the disease.

Rapid strides are being made, with powerful new methods leading us closer to understanding causes and mechanisms.[16] It is exciting that we are closing in on accurate PET and spinal tap markers for Alzheimer's, but it will probably take at least five years before we have a test accurate enough to rely on. When that happens MND will make sense as a new diagnosis, but not before. Let's not jump the gun, proceeding on the false belief that a diagnostic breakthrough has already been made and that a treatment breakthrough is possible in the near future. Without a laboratory test, the diagnosis of MNCD will be wildly inaccurate, pulling in many people who are not headed for dementia. And what purpose is served by revealing the early stages of a grim disease for which there is no meaningful treatment?[17] Finding out that you are (only possibly) at risk for later developing Alzheimer's would provide little or no benefit—but would create needless worry, testing, treatment, expense, stigma, and insurance and disability issues.

We also shouldn't oversell the prospects of any immediate treatment breakthrough. Learning more about the mechanisms of Alzheimer's may quickly lead to a rational cure or preventive—but more likely it won't. The general experience in medicine over the past three decades is that an exponential explosion in knowledge about a disease does not often lead to any immediate miracle cure. The lack of success in developing medications for Alzheimer's does not inspire confidence.[18] The available drugs—although they have been highly profitable to the drug companies—have little, if any, efficacy for patients. Attempts to develop a new generation of effective drugs have failed despite considerable research investment. There does not appear to be any low-hanging fruit.

The experts on Alzheimer's have a natural enthusiasm for pushing the boundaries toward earlier diagnosis. The slow pace of development of diagnostic and treatment tools is frustrating for all concerned. Most of us expected well-established laboratory testing by now and are very disappointed that drug discovery has been such a flop. MCND is offered in the hope it will jump-start the field by highlighting the potential of early identification. But this is definitely putting the cart before horse. New diagnoses that will have great influence on how people live their lives and how the country will spend limited health care dollars must follow well-established science and an inclusive public policy debate—not lead it.

The experts suggesting MNCD are acting from naive good faith that expanding their field will be good for patients. They are blind to false positive risks and societal costs because they are not trained to think in these terms, not because of conflicts of interest. But such goodwill does not motivate the corporations that market drugs and diagnostic tests. If MCND becomes official, there will be an explosion of probably useless and potentially harmful PET and spinal tap testing and medication treatment. The medical-industrial complex will have a field day.[19] Only they will benefit, not patients and not taxpayers.

Gluttony Becomes Mental Illness

I meet the criteria for binge eating disorder and have for almost as long as I can remember. It started in my early teenage years. Stealth trips to my mother's overly stocked pantry and bulging refrigerator leading to solitary nighttime pig-outs of epic proportions. In college, I wrestled at 177 pounds but after the match would begin a two-day binge that would bring me up to a Monday weight of 191—and would then have to starve and dehydrate to get back to 177 by the next Saturday. I have always been the scourge of buffet lines and all-you-can-eat restaurants. Never have I gone for more than a week without a monster binge. The only way I can stay a svelte twenty-five pounds overweight is to avoid all breakfasts and lunches and by exercising several hours a day. Am I just a run-of-the-mill glutton with terrible eating habits and lousy self-control or am I a *DSM-5* mental patient with binge eating disorder?

Certainly, I am not alone. BED would be a very low threshold diagnosis. Just one binge a week for only three months and you qualify for this alleged mental illness. The early estimate is that BED would capture about 3 to 5 percent of the population, but early estimates are always far too low.[20] Just wait until the public and the doctors get their drug-company-sponsored "education" selling the notion that glut-, tony (once a sin) has now become an illness. Rates may jump to 10 percent—adding twenty million fake mental patients in the U.S. alone.

Why do I binge eat? Why does anyone? Nature made it so. Our appetites are perfectly designed to ride out famine, but they make us terribly vulnerable to feast. When food was hard to come by, the best bet for survival was to be the biggest binger at the carcass. The availability of refrigerators and cheap fast food has certainly made binging a huge health risk—but I don't see how this makes it a mental disorder.

BED is being offered as psychiatry's answer to the obesity epidemic (which is rapidly overtaking smoking as our most deadly public health threat). Unfortunately psychiatry has no answers here—no cure for binge eating or for obesity. But even more to the point, BED distracts attention from what could provide a real cure for the obesity epidemic. We need a dramatic change in public policy. Our society is getting way too fat not because of an epidemic of this newly devised mental disorder, but rather through the ever present and always tempting availability of cheap, delicious, convenient, caloric, and horribly unhealthy fast food, snacks, and sodas. To make matters worse, we perversely incentivize this public health time bomb with government subsidies to Big Agriculture. For hundreds of thousands of years, until just three hundred years ago, the average person rarely if ever got to taste anything sweet. Then sugar entered our lives, and now fructose, and we are being fattened like cattle on a feedlot.

Mental disorder is not causing the obesity epidemic. And treating a fake mental disorder can't fix it. It won't help to label as psychiatrically sick the victims of our dumb public policies; it's far better to change the policies. No more fructose subsidies. No more Coke and fries served with school lunches. No more streets without sidewalks that discourage walking. Let's restore physical education in the schools; add calorie counts to every menu; subsidize vegetables; give people tax deductions and lower insurance premiums for losing weight; install free bikes at stands in cities everywhere. In short, we need to do whatever it takes from a public policy standpoint to encourage people to eat less and exercise more.

Phony psychiatric labels won't help. BED has the familiar three-strikes-you're-out combination of inaccurate diagnosis, no effective treatment, and drug side effects. Making BED focuses attention on the wrong culprit; it is not the individual who is sick, it is the public policy. We need to change attitudes about eating and exercise with the same total push educational campaign that worked so well to contain smoking.

Adult Attention-Deficit Hyperactivity Disorder Could Become the New Diagnosis du Jour

Unchastened by the false "epidemic" of ADHD already running rampant among kids, *DSM-5* has set the stage for creating a new epidemic of ADHD in adults. As usual, the experts worry so much about missed cases, they fail to consider the much greater risk of overdiagnosis. Attentional problems and restlessness are nonspecific and extremely common among normal adults and in those suffering from any of the other mental disorders. The easy path to adult ADHD suggested by *DSM-5* will mislabel many normal people who are dissatisfied with their ability to concentrate and get their work done, especially when they feel bored and don't like the work they're doing. It will also misdiagnose those whose problem in concentrating is really caused by something else—e.g., substance abuse, bipolar disorder, depression, all the anxiety disorders, OCD, autistic disorders, psychotic disorders, and many others. No one should ever get diagnosed or treated for adult ADHD until all of these are first ruled out as the primary cause—lest inappropriate stimulant treatment may worsen their already existing psychiatric problems.[21]

Adult ADD is already too easily diagnosed. Perceived difficulties with attention and concentration abound, especially among perfectionists and those over fifty. Symptoms are mostly subjective, based on fallible self-perceptions of poor concentration and task accomplishment. The *DSM-5* lowering of requirements will capture many adults who want to be sharper but don't have specific or serious enough problems to qualify for a mental disorder. Fake adult ADHD will also be especially common in college students, in people who have demanding jobs, and in those who have to struggle to stay awake, like long-haul truck drivers.

Stimulants are among the most effective and safe of medications in psychiatry when given under appropriate supervision for someone who is accurately diagnosed. But they can cause serious side effects in anyone and are especially harmful when taken by someone with another diagnosis that has been misidentified as ADHD (especially substance use or bipolar disorder). The increasing use of stimulants as performance enhancers or for recreation also creates a large and illegal secondary street market.[22]

I have often heard people say: "Why worry so much about the over-prescription of stimulants, since these are relatively safe medications that are helpful in promoting improved cognitive functioning even in those who do not have clear-cut ADHD." This is wrong for both individual and societal reasons. We have to consider the harm to people with psychiatric or medical problems worsened by stimulants. And do we want to further encourage the already rampant illegal diversion of prescription drugs for sale on the street?[23] The wider distribution of stimulants is simply too important a public health and public policy issue to have been decided as an unintended consequence of decisions made by a small group of *DSM-5* experts who are focused on their own narrow diagnostic question. I have no opinion on the interesting question of whether stimulant use should be allowed for performance enhancement in normals who want improved cognitive and physical functioning. But I am strongly opposed to lowering the criteria for adult ADHD in a way that indirectly promotes their fake "medical" use in those who don't really have a mental disorder.[24]

Others argue that an increasingly demanding society is exposing previously subclinical ADHD symptoms. As performance standards are ratcheted up and external stimulation becomes nonstop and blaring, previously well-adapted individuals with mild ADHD may now be reaching a clinically significant level of impairment that qualifies as a mental disorder and requires treatment. My point back is that the difficulties people have in meeting society's expectations should not all be labeled as mental disorders. Thirty percent of college students cannot suddenly have developed ADHD. When Major League Baseball finally controlled steroid use by testing, there was a sudden explosion of ADHD among the players—this was probably triggered more by a desire for improved batting averages than any of the traditional reasons for treating ADHD. If we, as a society, choose to help people enhance their performance to meet (perhaps excessive) demands, this should be an open policy decision—not one cloaked under medical auspices, done by medical prescription, and enhanced by drug company marketing.

The criteria for a first-time diagnosis of ADHD in adults should be more, not less, rigorous. In evaluating any given adult for ADHD, we must be sure that all the many psychiatric causes of inattention are first ruled out and that the problems are a continuation of ADHD symptoms that started in early childhood. Any late onset of attentional problems is caused by something else, not ADHD. Let's keep *DSM* as a manual of mental disorders and not turn it into a vehicle for performance enhancement.

Mourning Is Confused with Melancholia

DSM-5 has made it easier to diagnose major depressive disorder (MDD) among the bereaved, even in the first weeks after their loss. This was a stubbornly misguided decision in the face of universal opposition from clinicians, professional associations and journals, the press, and hundreds of thousands of grievers from all around the world. People routinely have symptoms exactly like clinical depression as part of their normal mourning process. Feeling sad, losing interest, trouble sleeping and eating, reduced energy, difficulty working—this is the easily recognizable, classic picture of grief. But these very same symptoms define clinical depression. MDD need not be diagnosed unless the bereaved becomes suicidal, or delusional, or suffers from symptoms that are severe, prolonged, and incapacitating.

Psychiatry should tread lightly when dealing with the basic rhythms of life. Mammals grieve. It is the flip side and necessary price of the quintessential mammalian characteristic—attachment to loved ones. We start life needing a mother not only for milk, but also for love. Our lives consist of a series of attachments and losses. And then we die and others grieve for us. Man is not alone as a caring and grieving social animal. We are just doing what mammals do.

Medicalizing grief reduces the dignity of the pain, short-circuits the expected existential processing of the loss, reduces reliance on the many well-established cultural rituals for consoling grief, and would subject grievers to unnecessary and potentially harmful medication. There is no uniform code of correct grieving. Different cultures prescribe a wide variety of time-honored behavioral and emotional reactions and rituals. Even within a given culture, normal individuals vary enormously in the content, symptoms, duration, and impairment of their grief and in their ability to draw consolation and sustenance from others.

There is no clear line separating those who are experiencing loss in their own necessary and particular way from those who will stay stuck in a depression unless they receive specialized psychiatric help. Except when the need is clear, psychiatry should not impose its own rituals when they are so often unneeded and out of place. The medicalization of grief sends just the wrong message to the misidentified "patient" and to the surviving family. To mislabel grief as a mental disorder reduces the dignity of the life lost and of the survivors' reactions to its loss. We would be substituting a half-baked, superficial, and depersonalizing medical mourning ritual for the solemn, time-tested death rituals that are at the heart of every culture. Most people will recover just fine after the loss, without medical meddling and pill popping.

There is a legitimate concern that major depression sometimes occurs among the bereaved. When a griever becomes suicidal, psychotic, agitated, or incapacitated, the diagnosis of depression is certainly warranted and treatment should begin immediately. People with a previous history of depression are at high risk for recurrence and should be followed expectantly and treated promptly. But these are exceptions. Grief is part of life, and most people work through it best with family and cultural supports, not psychiatric diagnosis and treatment.[25, 26, 27, 28, 29]

Turning Our Passions into Addictions

This actually happened today, just a few hours ago. I was walking up the hill, head buried in my BlackBerry, thumb thumping away e-mail responses, guided by my wife to avoid cars and obstacles, stumbling only occasionally over tree roots. It was an absolutely gorgeous Indian summer day, and my beloved beach and ocean would be clearly visible on all sides if only I bothered to look up. But I am head down, fully absorbed, totally oblivious, blind to everything but tiny keyboard and screen. Along comes a guy approaching quickly from the opposite direction, and we almost crash into each other. I quickly apologize. But he smiles sympathetically and says, "No problem, I understand— 'Crackberry' addict, huh?" I smile back sheepishly and then quickly return to my thumping.

Guilty as charged. You know you are busted and badly hooked when everybody calls your cell phone the "crackberry." Me hunched intently over my BlackBerry reminds people of King Kong playing with his cute pocket-size playmate. And I don't want to get too intimate here, but my wife does express feelings of jealousy and chagrin that she is forced to play second fiddle to what she calls "your mistress."

Is this mental disorder or just my avid utilization of a remarkably versatile device? "Behavioral addiction" or "BlackBerry affection"? Up

until now this was no more than a lame joke, but it's now a dead serious problem since *DSM-5* has introduced the concept of "behavioral
addictions." [30] For starters, only pathological gambling will qualify as
an official mental disorder. But watch out for false epidemics of addictions to the Internet,[31] shopping,[32] working,[33] sex, golf, jogging,[34] tanning,[35] model railroads, cleaning house, cooking, gardening, watching
sports on TV, surfing, or chocolate,[36] or whatever else commands passionate interest and media attention. The list is long and can easily
expand into every area of popular activity, turning lifestyle choices
into mental disorders.

The rationale for this radical proposal is that compulsive behavior
is equivalent to compulsive substance use and is caused by the same
brain pleasure centers—an interesting idea for research, but way premature to justify a huge expansion of psychiatric diagnosis.

The term "addiction" is being stretched to include any passionate
interest or attachment. It was once narrowly restricted to describe physical dependence on a substance or alcohol—you needed more and more
to get high and had painful withdrawal symptoms when you stopped.
Then "addiction" was expanded to cover compulsive substance use. The
addict is someone who feels compelled to take the drug even though it
no longer makes any sense. The fun is gone and there are grave negative
consequences, but he is driven to continue. Lately, "addiction" is loosely
and incorrectly applied to any frequent drug use—even if it is purely for
pleasurable recreational purposes, not yet compulsive. *DSM-5* takes the
final broadening step that we are just as addicted to our favorite behaviors as someone who is hooked on opium.

The concept of "behavioral addiction" has the fundamental flaw
that we are all "behavioral addicts." Repetitive pleasure seeking is part
of human nature and too common to be considered a mental disorder. Millions of new "patients" might be created by fiat, medicalizing all manner of passionate interests and giving people a "sick role"
excuse for their impulsive hedonism. I can picture the caption of the
New Yorker cartoon: "Sorry, honey, I just couldn't resist (you fill in the

blank). Doc says it's not my fault—I'm addicted." Individual accountability may never survive the shock.

We are all ruled by short-term brain pleasure centers that favor
our immediate survival or the survival of our DNA into the next generation. This is why it is so difficult for people to control impulses
toward food and sex, especially when the modern world provides such
tempting opportunities for both. The evolution of our brains was
strongly influenced by the fact that, until recently, most people did not
live very long. Given our lengthened life spans, longer term planning
has become the much better bet, but instincts don't change quickly,
and balancing short-term gains against long-term consequences just
doesn't come very naturally to most people. Our pleasure systems are
still responding to the world of our ancestors and often cause us trouble in our current world.

The proper and narrow definition of the term "behavioral addiction" would reserve it only for those who experience an override in
this average expectable pleasure system—who do the behavior over
and over and over and over again, despite the lack of even short-term
reward and in the face of extremely negative short-term punishments
(financial devastation, loss of family, jail). Such a negative reward/risk
ratio does not now (and never could have had) any survival value and
rightly might be considered a mental disorder. "Behavioral addiction"
might be a viable concept if it could be contained within the confines
of this very narrow definition. It is instead a terrible idea precisely because it would quickly spread far beyond its proper narrow confines.
Compulsive, nonpleasurable repetition is very difficult (or impossible)
to distinguish from impulsive self-indulgence.

"Addiction" should be reserved for those who feel compelled to
keep repeating the act even when the fun has worn off and the cost
is so high that no reasonable person would pay it. But how to tell
the difference between this and pleasure seeking? "Behavioral addiction" will undoubtedly expand to become the excuse du jour for
all impulsive behaviors that have gotten someone into any sort of

trouble. The twelve steps will substitute for the religious rituals of confession and expiation. Sometimes accepting that you are powerless over the "behavioral addiction" will be the beginning of a sincere effort to change, but often it will be no more than spin. A vibrant society depends on having responsible citizens who feel in control of themselves and own up to the consequences of their actions—not an army of "behavioral addicts" who need therapy in order to learn to do the right thing.

We had a parallel discussion whether caffeine dependence should be included as an official category in *DSM-IV*. Caffeine is as addictive as nicotine, can cause intoxication, and can provoke anxiety disorder and cardiac problems. We left it out for one reason only. Caffeine dependence is so ubiquitous (and mostly harmless) that it did not seem worthwhile to have sixty million people wake up each day to the awareness that their morning pleasure was a mental disorder. Similar constraint and caution would lead to the rejection of the category "behavioral addiction." The fact that it would be so widely misapplied greatly overwhelms any benefit.

The most likely contender for imminent fad status is "Internet addiction." All the elements for wildfire spread are in place—the profusion of alarming books; the breathless articles in magazines and newspapers; extensive TV exposure; ubiquitous blogs; the springing up of unproven treatment programs; the availability of millions of potential patients; and an exuberant trumpeting by newly minted "thought leading" researchers and clinicians. *DSM-5* showed restraint, relegating Internet addiction to an obscure appendix rather than legitimizing it as an official psychiatric diagnosis. But watch for Internet addiction to pick up steam even without full *DSM-5* endorsement. Granted that lots of us are furtively checking e-mails in movie theaters and in the middle of the night, feel lost when temporarily separated from our electronic friends, and spend every spare minute surfing, texting, or playing games. But does this really qualify us as addicts? No, not usually. Not unless our attachment is compulsive and without reward or utility; interferes with participation and success in real life; and causes significant distress or impairment. For most people, the tie to the Internet, however powerful and consuming, brings much more pleasure or productivity than pain and impairment. This is more love affair and/or tool-using than enslavement—and is not best considered the stuff of mental disorder. It would be silly to define as psychiatric illness behavior that has now become so much a necessary part of everyone's daily life and work.

But what about the small minority of Internet users who really are stuck in a pattern of joyless, compulsive, worthless, and self-destructive use—the 24/7 gamers, the shut-ins, the people trapped in virtual lives. The concept of addiction may indeed apply to many of them, and diagnosis and treatment may someday prove useful. But not yet. We don't know how to define Internet addiction in a way that will not also mislabel the many who are doing just fine being chained to their electronics. We also don't know what proportion of excessive users is stuck on the Internet because they have another psychiatric problem that may be missed if Internet addiction becomes an explain-all masking underlying problems. So far, the research on "Internet addiction" is remarkably thin and not very informative. Don't get too excited by pretty pictures showing the same parts of the brain lighting up during Internet and drug use—they light up nonspecifically for any highly valued activity and are not indicative of pathology. "Internet addiction" needs to be less a media darling, more a target of sober research. South Korea is the most wired country in the world and has the biggest problem with excessive Internet use. The government is attempting to tackle this with education, research, and intelligent public policy—none of which has required declaring "Internet addiction" a mental disorder. This is an excellent model for the rest of the world to follow.

Mislabeling Medical Illness as Mental Disorder

The boundary between psychiatry and medicine presents difficulties for both sides and is well served by neither. Even under the best of circumstances, the distinction between medical and psychiatric illness is often fuzzy and hard to draw. And it doesn't help that most medical doctors are not very expert at psychiatry and that most psychiatrists are not very expert about medical illness, and that the communication between the two specialties is often incomplete and/or confused. It is the patients who suffer, frequently falling through the cracks and getting second-rate care from both specialties.

I first became personally and painfully aware of the risks of misdiagnosis four decades ago when, as a brand-new psychiatric resident, I treated a man for what seemed to be depression for two months before discovering that his problems were in fact caused by the brain tumor I had previously missed. During the years since, I have seen in consultation dozens of patients who had a medical illness that had been previously mislabeled psychiatric and dozens of patients who had a psychiatric illness that had previously been mislabeled medical. It is easy to screw up in both directions.

There are four ways mistakes are made. First, some medical illnesses present with severe physical symptoms, but no definitive pathology (typical examples are irritable bowel, chronic fatigue, fibromyalgia, chronic pain, Lyme disease, and interstitial cystitis). Too often the patients are told that it is all in their heads and are called "crocks" behind their backs, thus adding insult to the injury and impairment of their chronic and sometimes debilitating illness.

Second, medical illnesses may present with symptoms that go unexplained for many years before the underlying cause clearly declares itself. Typical examples are multiple sclerosis, lupus, rheumatoid arthritis, peripheral neuropathies, connective tissue diseases, and yes, brain tumors. Uncertainty is hard to live with, but much better than jumping to the false and risky conclusion that the problem is psychiatric.

Third, some people have very strong psychological reactions to their cancer or heart disease or diabetes or other serious illness. And why not? When you are sick, it is understandable that you may become worried about your health, preoccupied with efforts to improve it, and hyperalert to possible new symptoms. That seemingly run-of-the-mill headache could always be a recurrence of brain tumor. People who have medical illnesses should not be casually mislabeled as also having a mental illness just because they are fearful and upset about being sick.

Fourth, the mislabeling also goes in the opposite direction. Many psychiatric disorders present with prominent somatic symptoms that are often mistaken for medical illness. The best example: People with panic attacks typically get far too much unnecessary, costly, and potentially harmful medical testing for the dizziness, shortness of breath, and palpitations that are really just part of the hyperventilation caused by the panic. And depression sometimes also presents with prominent somatic symptoms, especially weight loss.

DSM-5 will make even fuzzier the already fuzzy boundary between medical and mental illness by introducing a new diagnosis, "somatic symptom disorder," and providing it with a loose and easy-to-meet definition. The result will be dramatically increased rates of mental disorder in all three patient groups: people whose diseases have clearly defined pathology (like cancer); people whose diseases have less well understood causes (like fibromyalgia); and people whose physical symptoms are thus far unexplained but will later show a clear etiology (like multiple sclerosis).

The often incorrect diagnosis of mental disorder will be based solely on the clinician's subjective and fallible judgment that the patient's life has become subsumed with health concerns and preoccupations, or that the response to distressing somatic symptoms is excessive or disproportionate, or that the coping strategies to deal with the symptom are maladaptive. These are inherently unreliable and un-trustworthy assessments that will open the floodgates to the overdiagnosis of mental disorder and result in the missed diagnosis of medical disorder.

DSM-5's own field trials produced pretty scary results. One in six cancer and coronary disease patients met the criteria for *DSM-5* "somatic symptom disorder." So did one in four patients with irritable bowel syndrome or fibromyalgia. And get this: so did almost one in ten "healthy" people. Do we really want to so casually burden medically ill (and even healthy) people with an additional diagnosis of mental illness just because they are worried about being sick?

An incautious, inept misapplication of *DSM-5*'s highly subjective and catch-all criteria will likely result in frequent inappropriate psychiatric diagnosis with far-reaching implications. Possible harms include:

- Stigma
- Missed medical diagnoses through failure to investigate new or worsening somatic symptoms
- Disadvantages in getting or keeping a job
- Reduced medical and disability reimbursement
- Reduced eligibility for social, medical, and education services and workplace accommodations
- A reluctance on the part of patients with life-threatening diseases to report new symptoms that might be early indicators of recurrence, metastasis, or secondary illness for fear of attracting a mental disorder diagnosis
- The patient's view of herself and her illness may be skewed, as are the perceptions of family and friends
- The prescription of inappropriate psychotropic drugs

The burden of the DSM-5 changes will fall mostly on women because they are more likely to be casually dismissed when presenting with physical symptoms and also are more likely to receive inappropriate antidepressants and antianxiety medications.

The golden rules: An underlying medical illness has to be ruled out before ever deciding that someone's symptoms are caused by a mental disorder. People suffering from a medical illness should never be casually mislabeled as also being mentally ill just because they are upset about being sick. And finally, there is lots of uncertainty inherent in determining whether a physical symptom springs from a physical or an emotional cause or has elements of both. Much better to live with the uncertainty than to mislabel psychiatric diagnosis.

Dodged Bullets—But Still Beware

This section describes the proposed disorders that almost made it into *DSM-5* but got scrubbed at the very last moment. A big relief—none is remotely ready for prime time. But careful vigilance against their fad use is still required. Childhood bipolar disorder was similarly rejected by *DSM-IV* but nonetheless managed to become a dangerous false epidemic. And Australia is about to embark on a nationwide program, spending almost half a billion dollars, to treat psychosis risk—even though it is not an official diagnosis.

Psychosis Risk Is Far Too Risky

The future is good at keeping secrets and very hard to predict. Particularly with teenagers, who often seem like strangers in a strange land—or perhaps like Alice in Wonderland. The metamorphosis from child to adult has too many puzzling things happening far too fast—body changes, sexual maturation, new roles, new ideas, new feelings, new relationships, new responsibilities, new freedoms, new temptations. Teenagers confront the world fresh, asking unsettling

questions that grown-ups know have no answers. They worry about
the meaning of life and the mysteries of the universe, often speaking in abstract ways that befuddle busy parents worried about the
next mortgage payment. Teenagers are not comfortable in their own
skin—their sense of identity is fragile, uncertain, and unstable. Existential fears abound, fantasies are weird, feelings extreme, self-esteem
shaky, dress eccentric, behavior erratic, video game play constant.
Taste in music, movies, pastimes—all are likely to be abominable.
It's easy for teenagers to feel persecuted, insulted, ganged up against,
and misunderstood. They are needy but reject help. Kindly concern is
misunderstood as hostile intrusiveness. Parents are often at their wit's
end in trying to understand their previously loving child and imagine
the worst for the future.

All of the above gets even more complicated when the troubled
teen starts using drugs. The more troubled the teen, the more likely
and the heavier will be the usage. The difficulties and confusions of
growing up are magnified by mind-altering drugs that have the capacity to mimic every psychiatric condition. Some drugs create a particular good imitation of prepsychotic or psychotic symptoms—seeing
or hearing things that aren't there, developing strange beliefs that approach the delusional, becoming paranoid and hypervigilant, losing
motivation, neglecting responsibilities and personal hygiene, and entering into weird countercultures. Under the influence of drugs, eccen-
tricities will be accentuated, thoughts fragmented, beliefs confused,
bizarre ideas accepted as plausible. Parents usually are either unin-
formed completely or greatly underestimate the role of the substance
in making their kids even weirder than they were before. The natural
fear is that one's child is going nuts.

The good news is that being a teenager is usually a self-and-time-
limited disease. Most troubled teens grow up to be normal adults. The
bad news is that some don't—their teenage problems just a prelude
for later continuing life difficulties. The worst news is that about one
percent of all teenagers will develop schizophrenia, a serious psychi-

atric illness characterized by psychotic delusions, hallucinations, and strange thinking and behavior. Great suffering would be avoided if only we could identify those at risk for schizophrenia and intervene early before they have experienced their first full-blown psychotic episode. Not only would this avoid tremendous short-term disruption, but it might also greatly improve the person's lifelong prospects. Preventing psychotic episodes is a high priority for psychiatry, a major preoccupation of the field for more twenty years. But how do you find the needle in the haystack—the rare strange teenager who will go on to be psychotic from the many other strange teenagers who will grow up to be normal?

DSM-5 proposed a new diagnosis intended to take on this daunting task. It has gone by two different names: "psychosis risk syndrome" and the tongue-twisting "attenuated psychotic symptoms syndrome." However named, the high-minded goal is to promote early identification and treatment—to help prevent the onset of schizophrenia, or at least to reduce its lifetime ravages. This effort, were it successfully accomplished, would be the highest achievement in the history of psychiatry. The ambition is to do a very great good, but the risk is that early identification will miss its mark and instead inflict a very great harm.

Good intentions are not good enough; you have to have good tools. The value of early intervention to prevent psychosis rests on three fundamental and necessary pillars—diagnosing only the right people, having a treatment that is effective, and also safe. Psychosis risk syndrome (PRS) strikes out badly on all three counts. It would misidentify many teenagers who are not really at risk for psychosis. They would often receive atypical antipsychotic medications that have no proven efficacy. And most damning, these drugs have extremely dangerous complications.

First, let's deal with the misidentification problem. Even in the most expert hands (i.e., in very highly selected research clinics), at least two of three people who get the PRS diagnosis do not go on to become psychotic. Of great counterintuitive interest, the longer the research clinic operates, the worse its correct hit rate. This doesn't mean the evaluators get dumber. It's just that, with time and spreading reputation, the clinic attracts an increasingly heterogeneous pool of referrals, so it becomes more difficult to pick out the needle of those truly at risk for psychosis from the haystack of those who aren't.

In the real world, the ratio gets really ridiculous: nine misses for every hit. The raters in general practice are much less expert than specialists in research clinics, and the "patients" are closer to normal and harder to discriminate. Mislabeling may get even worse if the diagnosis ever becomes official and drug companies get into the act, trying to convince parents and clinicians to be especially alert to any strangeness in teenagers.[37,38,39,40]

Kids not really at high risk for psychosis would often receive a preventive medication treatment that puts them at high risk for obesity and diabetes and all the dreaded health consequences that follow.[41] To top it all off, there is no proof whatever that antipsychotic medications are effective in preventing psychotic episodes.

It gets even worse. The terms "psychosis risk" and "attenuated psychotic symptoms syndrome" are filled with ominous threat and undeniable stigma. The mislabeled person bears the needless cross of unnecessary worry, reduced ambitions, and likely discrimination in getting work or insurance or a mate—thus further exacerbating the risk side of the already totally unbalanced risk-benefit ratio.

So let's add up the score: most kids who get tagged with PRS are not really at risk for psychosis; the preventive treatment they will very often get doesn't really prevent, but will likely make them fat and reduce their life expectancy; and the label is itself a new life burden. This is a prescription for individual tragedy and public health disaster.

Mixed Anxiety/Depression—Turning Everyone into a Patient

DSM-5 proposed a new disorder that would have been the darling of diagnostic inflation and the greatest gift ever to the drug companies. The criteria set was so easy to make that sooner or later virtually everyone would wind up qualifying for it. Mixed anxiety depression (MAD) is perhaps the most flagrant attempt ever to medicalize the transient, nonspecific, almost ubiquitous sadness and worries that are an inevitable part of everyday life. A perfectly expectable reaction to bad events—job loss, divorce, illness, or financial troubles—would have been converted into mental disorder. Not surprisingly, MAD is an unstable diagnosis that provides little predictive power. Studied a year later, most people tagged with it either will have gotten over their symptoms and need no diagnosis at all or will have evolved into another more established diagnosis. Watchful waiting is the wiser and safer course, rather than jumping the gun to what is an essentially meaningless diagnosis.

The only thing about MAD that is absolutely predictable is its huge marketing potential. Turning life's inevitable problems into mental disorder would have been an absolute gold mine for the drug companies—the perfect combination of huge market share and high placebo response. Overnight, MAD would have emerged from nowhere to become the most common mental disorder in America. Antidepressants, already used by 11 percent of the population, would have gotten another big boost. Sanity finally prevailed on this one and MAD was shelved—but just barely.[42,43]

Hebephilia Creates a Constitutional Crisis

"Hebephilia" is a fancy medical-sounding term dreamed up more than a century ago as a parallel to pedophilia. Pedophiles are those who prefer or need prepubescent children in order to get sexually excited; in alleged "hebephiles" the preferential lust would be for teenagers who have already entered puberty.

Hebephilia has never caught on as a clinical entity and has generated almost no research. But it has become very popular as a fake diagnosis used in sexually violent predator (SVP) hearings to justify preventive detention through involuntary psychiatric commitment. This public safety convenience represents an abuse of psychiatry that violates precious constitutional guarantees against double jeopardy. *DSM-5* unwisely considered including hebephilia as an official diagnosis but wisely dropped it in response to the almost unanimous opposition of sexual disorder and forensic experts. Support for the inclusion of "hebephilia" came only from the handful of people who research it and the somewhat larger group of SVP evaluators who make part or all of their living misdiagnosing it.

Sex with an underage, pubescent teenager is a despicable crime deserving imprisonment, not a mental disorder treatable in a hospital. There is nothing inherently psychiatric about being sexually attracted to budding teenagers. Numerous studies have proven the obvious— such attraction is common and completely within the range of normal male lust. The age of condoned sexual activity has varied widely across different times and places, with puberty often taken as nature's dividing line to signify sexual eligibility. Until a hundred years ago, the age of consent was thirteen in the United States; it remains low in many parts of the developing world and has been raised only recently in much of the Western world.

Evolution has built teenage sexual attractiveness into male hardwiring. When our lives were much shorter and likely to end unpredictably at any moment, it made sense for our DNA to seek expression as soon as sexual maturation made this at all possible. Waiting patiently on the sexual sidelines entailed a great risk of losing out in the mating game. Remember the startling fact that the average age when people died is now the average age when people get married.

Optimal mating strategies have changed dramatically in response to longer life expectancy and lower infant mortality. If you are likely to live to seventy, there is no advantage to starting early on the path of sex and child rearing. There will be plenty of time; and both activities are safer and more wisely done as one matures. The legal age of consent has accordingly risen to protect youngsters from what is now regarded as premature sexual activity, given the conditions and expectations that prevail in our society.

But that doesn't mean that sexual wiring has caught up. Changes in basic appetites require evolutionary time frames of at least tens or hundreds of thousands of years; changes in laws can happen overnight. We don't turn off long-established instincts just because they are no longer considered proper. The advertising industry, wise to the fact that many adults remain sexually attracted to adolescents, cynically exploits their interest by displaying young-looking models in provocative clothing and poses. The assertion that sexual urges stimulated by sexy teenagers denote mental disorder violates common sense, experience, and evidence from research. It is not a crime or a mental disorder to lust after the newly pubescent; it is human nature. But it is a very serious crime in our society to act on these impulses, one that deserves a long prison term.

The only rationale for having a diagnosis of "hebephilia" might be to describe those rare individuals who are obsessively, exclusively, and obligatorily stuck just on very young teenagers. But the many compelling reasons for not including the diagnosis in *DSM-5* far outweighed this one possibly positive use. Hebephilia (if it exists at all) is unresearched; we have no idea how best to diagnose it and whether there is any effective treatment. There is no apparent clinical need for this proposed diagnosis—no army of help-seeking potential perpetrators willing and able to benefit from treatment, presuming one were available. And the careless forensic overuse in the SVP mill is already a serious problem. True hebephiles would constitute only a tiny fraction of all the criminals who violate the young. Experience teaches that this would not stop forensic evaluators from spreading the diagnosis widely and inappropriately as a lubricant to involuntary commitment in SVP hearings.

No tears need be shed for child molesters. But we lose constitutional stability whenever we allow civil rights to be violated, even for those people we most detest. If having sex with a teenager today constitutes mental disorder, what prevents future slippage in a possibly less enlightened time to revisit whether homosexuality isn't a mental disorder, or the use of psychiatry to suppress political dissent or minority religious belief. Whatever tiny clinical utility there might be for "hebephilia" is overwhelmed by its fearsome forensic risks.[44, 45, 46]

Hypersexuality—"My Disorder Made Me Do It"

This was another unwise proposal for *DSM-5*. Fortunately, it was rejected, but unfortunately it remains very much alive in the media and public consciousness. The most recognizable prototypes for excessive sexuality come from the worlds of professional sports, rock music, Hollywood, and politics. The term might cover previous presidents in the United States and Italy as well as powerful leaders in business and government. Whether it is Mickey or Wilt or Magic or Tiger or Silvio or JFK or the local Don Juan, the script is the same. The man (only rarely a woman) can't seem to get enough sex. Wilt Chamberlain boasted of sleeping with twenty thousand different women. A reporter ran the numbers and told Wilt this would amount to an average of about three a day. Wilt grinned, stroked his chin, and said, "Yup, that sounds about right."

The lack of consensus on what is normal sexual behavior makes it difficult to define what is excessive. Individual and cultural biases play a large role and offer a moving target. What is completely normal in New York or Amsterdam may not be at all accepted in Topeka or Mecca. What is normal in New York today was deviant in New York a century ago. What is normal for professional athletes may not be normal for the rest of us. There is tremendous variability and no clear standard. A lot may depend on opportunity.

Sexual excess is often misguided but rarely indicative of mental disorder. Humans, especially males, cheat so often it might almost be considered normative behavior, not sickness. Sex is so pleasurable precisely because our DNA totally depends on it for survival. Evolution has wired our brains to do what it takes to get our sperm and eggs into the next generation. Considerations of love, morality, loyalty, and long-term consequence often get swamped by low resistance to temptation.

In the evolutionary numbers game, people with a high sex drive tend to have more kids. Giving in to sexual temptation has strong survival value for our DNA—that's why we do it. This is perhaps regrettable, but it is how natural selection works, an expectable part of normal life—not mental disorder. The genes of Genghis Khan won the evolutionary crapshoot, living on in millions of modern-day descendants. The sexually meek do not inherit the earth.

The medicalization of sexual misbehavior is a serious mistake—reducing the culprit's sense of individual responsibility and providing an inappropriate psychiatric excuse for hedonism.[47]

From Diagnostic Inflation to Diagnostic Hyperinflation

Just as it is unwise to add to the money supply when there is already a monetary inflation, it is unwise to coin new diagnoses when there is already a glut of diagnostic inflation. DSM-5 failed to understand the need for restraint and instead will be triggering a whole new batch of unfortunate fads on top of the ones we already have. This will open the floodgates even wider to permit ever looser diagnosis and increasingly inappropriate treatment.[48] In a reasonable world, DSM-5 would have tacked in just the opposite direction to contain diagnostic inflation and to restrict treatment to situations where it is really needed. The

DSM-5 damage is done and cannot easily be undone. Perhaps the only solace is that the controversy surrounding *DSM-5* has widely discredited it, raising concerns about the harms done by diagnostic inflation. Many clinicians will see through *DSM-5*, will not give it undeserved "biblical" authority, and will perhaps be more cautious in diagnosis and prescribing. And many potential patients have been put on alert not to accept diagnoses that may make no sense for them.

PART III

Getting Back to Normal

CHAPTER 7

Taming Diagnostic Inflation

*For every complex problem there is an answer that is clear,
simple, and wrong.*
H. L. Mencken

Diagnostic inflation has many complex and interacting causes; solving it will require many, complex, and interacting cures—and the result is very much in doubt. What needs to be done is completely obvious, but having brains enough to know what to do is worthless without the muscle to do it. Most of the political and financial muscle is pushing abnormal; the counterbalancing forces pushing normal don't remotely counterbalance and aren't nearly forceful enough. But hope sometimes redeems itself. The meek occasionally do inherit the earth, especially if right is on their side. Unforeseen social and public health miracles can occur when no one could guess they were even remotely possible. Against all odds, we have elected a black president, passed gay marriage bills, and transformed smoking from a display of sexy sophistication into a dirty little habit. So who says we can't also tame the beast of diagnostic inflation and save the world from the epidemic spread of ubiquitous psychiatric illness. Here's how to do it.

We Are Fighting the Wrong War on Drugs

For forty years, we have been fighting a war against drug cartels that we can't possibly win. Meanwhile, we have barely begun to fight a different war against the misuse of legal drugs that we couldn't possibly lose.

Interdiction of street drugs now is as big a bust as prohibition of alcohol was in the 1920s.[1] Occasionally arresting a drug kingpin or confiscating a few million dollars' worth of contraband heroin or cocaine or amphetamines makes for a nice headline, but it doesn't do anything to stop the flow. The price of illegal drugs remains pretty constant and is never high enough to drive away the market. New sources are always ready to fill in for the odd missed shipment. However impressive the street value of the confiscated drugs, incredible quantities of drugs are always seeping through. Usage patterns aren't significantly impacted by even the biggest drug bust, making the whole drug interdiction campaign no more than a phony Whac-A-Mole charade.

Similarly insignificant are ballyhooed reports of the spectacular arrests or the deaths of high-level drug kingpins. This also never significantly affects street availability and instead causes a mostly negative cascade of side effects from the fierce turf battles that inevitably ensue. The end result is more killing and more corruption, not less drug use. The drug trade is extremely well organized and rationally run—as would be expected of any large, immensely profitable, multinational business enterprise. It follows business models and corporate structures similar to its competitors in the licit drug industry. The success of companies like Pfizer or Eli Lilly or Jansen is not dependent on who happens to be the current CEO. They have built-in operating procedures and infrastructure that govern business decisions and ensure continuity and enduring profits regardless of who happens to be in charge at any given moment. The illegal drug trade is much more violent (and marginally more ruthless), but its administrative structures are equally effective in the long-term pursuit of profit. Chopping off one cartel head doesn't have more than a very temporary effect on its body—the drug trade is hydra headed, resilient, and competent. Ever more ruthless pretenders to the throne are never lacking.

The main effect of the war on drugs has been the unimaginable enrichment of the drug cartels. This provides them with the means and motivation to enter into a military and political arms race with one another and with official governments; to buy officials with gold and bully them with lead; and to destabilize failing countries in what are really ongoing civil wars.[2] We have repeatedly done the experiment and should by now accept the result. The war on drugs has been fought and the war on drugs has been lost. If we continue to fight it, we will continue to lose it.

We have to address the fact that the misuse of legal drugs has now become a bigger public health problem than street drugs. It is unacceptable that 7 percent of our population is addicted to prescription drugs and that fatal overdoses with them now exceed those caused by illegal drugs.[3] The legal products pushed by the Eli Lillys and the Pfizers have (when overdone) become more dangerous than the street drugs pushed by the cartel corner boys. Our policy decisions haven't confronted this remarkable public health and public policy paradox. We are spending a fortune fighting the losing war against illegal drugs, while barely lifting a finger to fight an easily winnable war against the misuse of legal drugs.[4]

The good news is that the legal drug lords are extremely vulnerable to the law in ways that the illegal are not. They would be easy to control if only we had the political will to control them. Eli Lilly, AstraZeneca, Jansen, Abbott, Purdue et al. have the great advantage over the Sinaloa, Tijuana, and Juárez cartels that they can operate within the law and enjoy its protections. They can market (i.e., "push") product openly using TV, Internet, and print advertising;[5] distribute it cheaply through doctors and pharmacies; buy politicians legally through campaign contributions and revolving door jobs.[6] They need not fear being arrested by the police or being assassinated by rival corporations. But their reliance on the law is also a weak point, making these legal drug pushers much more vulnerable to its reach. The law could overnight prohibit their questionable practices and end their worst depredations.

Curing drug-company-induced diagnostic inflation is not rocket science and doesn't require high-level skills in regulation, jurisprudence, or policing. The list of things that need to be done could not be more obvious or easier to enforce. But the first step has to be for politicians to "Just Say No" to the financial blandishments dangled by Big Pharma—massive campaign contributions and tempting future job offers.

Dismantling the Marketing Machine

The legal psychiatric drugs industry has thrived through the aggressive spread of misinformation. Big Pharma has almost unlimited financial resources, political punch, marketing prowess, and greed in the pursuit of new markets and bigger profits.[7] But all this could be reversed on a dime if politicians had the motivation to do so. None of the following policy changes would be hard to enforce. Most of them are already in place in the rest of the world and work well to better contain, if not entirely eliminate, the excessive use of prescription drugs.

FOURTEEN WAYS TO TAME PHARMA

- No more direct-to-consumer advertising on TV, in magazines, or on the Internet
- No more drug company–sponsored junkets, dinners, promotional gifts, or continuing medical education for doctors or medical students[8]
- No more financial support for medical professional organizations
- No more beautiful salespeople congregating in the doctors' waiting room

- No more free samples[9]
- No more off-label marketing[10]
- No more co-opting of thought leaders[11]
- No more drug company funding for the Food and Drug Administration
- Bigger fines and criminal penalties for malfeasance that are directed against the executives as well as the companies[12]
- Shortened patent protection for companies that break the law.
- No more financial aid for consumer advocacy groups[13]
- No more disease-awareness campaigns[14]
- No more unlimited and undisclosed contributions to politicians
- A three-year quarantine before politicians, staffers, and bureaucrats involved in setting or monitoring drug company regulations can join a drug company as officer or employee

We can't expect the drug companies to reform spontaneously. They simply have no motivation to change as long as the profits are pouring in and their shareholders are happy. Their corporate mission is to make as much money as possible. Despite whatever protestations are made to the contrary, serving the public weal is low on their list of priorities. The public has to be protected from misleading information and monopoly pricing. And having laws on the books is not enough to contain greed unless the financial costs of breaking them exceed the gain—or a few executives do some jail time. Pharma will gorge as much as it can for as long as it can until it is stopped from without. Other countries do a much better job of containing Pharma's excesses than we have, probably because money doesn't convert so readily into political power in most other democracies. The best hope of reform is sustained public outrage at being ripped off. As Abraham Lincoln said, "You can fool some of the people all of the time, and all of the people some of the time, but you can't fool all of the people all of the time."

Controlling Distribution: Borrowing Tips from MasterCard

Diagnostic inflation and polypharmacy go hand in hand and can be a lethal combination. How remarkable that so little is being done to stop this almost completely preventable cause of death and disability—especially since there is an easy technical fix to end the glut of dangerous overprescription.

Any time a suspicious purchase is charged to your credit card, it gets picked up immediately and your card is temporarily suspended until the purchase is approved by you. This sometimes annoyingly efficient system is triggered if, for instance, you try to use your card in a foreign country without first having informed MasterCard that you are traveling. Why isn't a similarly efficient and proactive, real-time alert system in place to help control the rampant overprescription and overdispensing of psychotropic and pain medicines? If we have the technology to prevent a hundred-dollar fraud, it is silly not to apply it to prevent deaths from overdose with prescription drugs.

The distribution of illegal drugs has proven to be impossible to control despite determined and expensive law enforcement efforts at the borders and on the streets. The distribution of prescription drugs is a cinch to control because they are dispensed by pharmacies that could be linked by all-seeing computers. Guidelines could be established to tag all suspicious transactions (e.g., too many different drugs prescribed in tandem, or doses that are too high, or prescriptions that are filled too often and/or come from different doctors) and to identify doctors in the habit of serial overprescribing. If there was a good rationale for a given outlier, it would be allowed to go forward (equivalent to explaining to MasterCard the reason for the purchase that tickled their fraud alert). But potentially deadly drug cocktails and deadly doctors would be identified and stopped dead in their tracks.

I can think of only three possible objections, and none hold any water. The first is expense—who will pay for it? This is silly. We spend a fortune failing to interdict illegal drugs at the border because it is so impossible to seal. But our pharmacies, equivalent to the border as distribution points for licit drugs, are easy and cheap to patrol with never-sleeping computers. It is also a no-brainer who should pay for the sentinel system—the monitoring money should come from a tiny tax on Pharma's gigantic drug revenue.

Second concern—how do we get all the drug companies and all the pharmacies to participate in such a system? Isn't the prescription and dispensing of medicine too fragmentary to allow for central control? Not at all. Pharmacy chains and large Internet mail-order delivery systems could easily be compelled to comply with a prescription drug abuse interdiction system.

The third objection is the only one with any merit: Isn't a warning system a potential Big Brother invasion of individual privacy that in the wrong hands could lead to abuses? This argument would have more traction if the need to protect from legal drug overdosing weren't so urgent and if privacy in prescribing wasn't already quite vulnerable, given the record-keeping and surveillance systems already in place. Adding a universal alarm system with teeth would provide enormous benefit, while incurring very little additional risk.

Would this have much impact on diagnostic inflation? Yes, because this tail wags the dog. Whenever a diagnosis is an easy ticket to getting a desired drug, it is made much more frequently. Loose diagnosing/high-prescribing doctors will tighten up on both counts when they know that the computer's eagle eye is fixed relentlessly upon them.

This is the one battle that the war against drugs can and should win.

Sunsetting Bad Drugs

The Food and Drug Administration goes to considerable (though not nearly sufficient) lengths to vet new drugs before they are approved for market. But once invited to the party, a drug gets pretty much a free ride for the rest of its life. Unless a drug is blatant in its complications or actually kills people, it is likely to fly under the radar for decades. The FDA's postapproval surveillance program is greatly underfunded and not up to the task of monitoring all the useless and/or harmful drugs that have made it to market.

Take Xanax. Introduced in the 1980s as a wonder drug to replace Valium and Librium, it is loved by patients and used frequently by primary care physicians. But Xanax has been more a wonder of profitability and longevity than a useful medication. Its therapeutic dosage is often high enough to be addicting, and its severe withdrawal anxiety is enough to keep patients hooked for life. Attempts at withdrawal may bring on severe panic or anxiety symptoms that are worse than the problems the patient started with.[15] Xanax is also a frequent collaborator with other prescription drugs and alcohol in iatrogenic overdoses and deaths.[16] It has little role, if any, in the proper practice of medicine. If there was a proper war against prescription drug misuse, Xanax would be an early casualty—but under current policies the FDA has no mechanism to rein in drugs that do more harm than good. We need a better way to identify and sunset bad drugs.

Taming the Doctors

Most doctors try to be responsible in the way they prescribe medication, but the few really bad apples can do a whole lot of damage. They are to the licit drug trade what the corner boy is to the illicit. It is extremely easy to identify these "highfliers" by medical monitoring and audit. They see the most patients for the shortest number of minutes. In the limited time allotted, they give the most psychiatric diagnoses—and often these are the same diagnoses and medications for every patient. They write the most prescriptions for multiple medications per patient at the highest average doses, and every patient may be on the same drug cocktail. They also probably charge the most per visit but may have trouble remembering the patient's name or problem. They attend drug company events religiously and may sometimes speak at them, extolling the latest new wonder drug. Their office is a magnet for drug salespeople, all of whom are on a chummy first-name basis with the secretary. The office is strewn with drug company presents and paraphernalia. Our highflier probably drives the best car and lives in the best house. Every so often, a patient dies of a drug overdose of the medicine he has prescribed (perhaps helped along a bit by alcohol), but he has never been disciplined, is a pillar of the professional community, and thinks highly of his or her clinical skills. (I have written another book, *Essentials of Psychiatric Diagnosis*, which provides tips to the accurate diagnosis of each of the mental disorders and cautions on how to avoid diagnostic inflation.)

The most primitive of computerized drug-monitoring systems can easily spot highfliers and brand them as dramatic outliers to proper medical practice. The most elementary of quality control measures would force them to justify their decisions, which immediately would take some of the wind out of their sails. Professional disciplining of one highflier would bring the others into line, and public shaming would ground them all. It can be done and would be done as part of a comprehensive War on Licit Drug Misuse. It is now being done almost not at all. Most medical corner boys ply their trade with impunity, and patients pay the price in disability, sometimes death. Improper polypharmacy could be stopped within months if proper monitoring and quality control were put in place.

Taming *DSM*

The loose *DSM* criteria that encourage diagnostic inflation need tightening. This won't be easy—the problem has taken thirty years to build up and has been aggravated by *DSM-5*. But errors do have a way of correcting with time, and now is the time to begin this correction. Thresholds for many existing diagnoses should be changed to require more symptoms and/or longer durations and/or more impairment.

And we need to stop adding new diagnoses unless there are very compelling reasons to do so.

DSM should also gradually be relieved of some of its responsibility, decoupling it from decisions that have been tied exclusively to the presence or absence of a psychiatric diagnosis. School services should be based on a thorough evaluation of educational need, not just on the presence or absence of a diagnosis. Autism and attention deficit disorder were defined for clinical, not educational, purposes and don't work very well as determinants of classroom decisions. Levels of educational impairment can vary very widely in people who have the same diagnosis. Similarly, eligibility for disability and other benefits should depend more on the person's actual level of functional impairment, less on whether or not he has a psychiatric diagnosis. And *DSM*s should not be relied on so heavily in legal proceedings.

Psychiatric diagnosis used to be just a modest clinical tool having little outside influence. Now that the reach of *DSM* has grown out of all proportion, it is the sole arbiter of all sorts of decisions not always within its competence. This adds more weight than the diagnostic system can comfortably carry and increases diagnostic inflation as clinicians up-diagnose their patients to get them added services and benefits. A less important *DSM* will be a better *DSM* and result in more accurate diagnosis.

Psychiatric Diagnosis Is Too Important to Be Left to the Psychiatrists

The American Psychiatric Association has held a guild monopoly on psychiatric diagnosis for the past century. This happened only by historical accident, not by design. Until 1980 and *DSM-III*, no one else much cared about *DSM*—its management was a burden that APA assumed only because it was too unimportant to warrant more official sponsorship. Things have since dramatically changed—psychiatric diagnosis has grown greatly in importance and the APA has shrunk in its competence.

DSM-5 has been the last straw and the loud wake-up call. The APA governance structure proved itself incapable of governance. Reckless changes suggested by researchers pushing their pet theories were insufficiently vetted for real world impact. Experts in clinical care, epidemiology, health economics, forensics, and public policy were left out of the loop. Decisions were mostly made by and for psychiatrists—ignoring the fact that they constitute only 7 percent of all mental health clinicians and now write only a small minority of prescriptions for all psychotropic drugs. APA has not acted as if *DSM-5* is a public trust, treating it instead like a publishing product and profit center.

The *DSM-5* follies prove that psychiatric diagnosis has outgrown APA—becoming too important in too many aspects of life to be left in the hands of one small professional organization with its limited skill set and no public accountability. Psychiatrists will always be an important part of the mix, but the APA should no longer be calling the shots. Its exclusive monopoly over psychiatric diagnosis should end now.

Next obvious question—if the APA has permanently disqualified itself as keeper of the flame, who should step in to mind it? Regrettably, no existing structure is ready to take on this responsibility. Psychiatric diagnosis should not become the monopoly of a different mental health association—the psychologists would muck it up just as badly (if in different ways). The National Institute of Mental Health has the resources, intellectual firepower, and moral authority, but its emphasis and expertise are increasingly focused almost exclusively on basic science research. NIMH has little concern about, or skill in, handling practical clinical questions. Its *DSM* would be a researcher's dream list but a nightmare for clinicians, patients, and public policy. The World Health Organization might be a contender, but its spotty past performance in producing its own manual of mental disorders does not inspire any great confidence. There are no other organizational structures off-the-shelf ready to fill the breach.

I think that psychiatric diagnosis requires and deserves its own new regulatory structure. The Food and Drug Administration is the closest existing model. This is not as far-fetched as it may seem. New diagnoses in psychiatry are potentially much more dangerous than new drugs because they can lead to massive overtreatment (with all the possible side effects), while new drugs are generally no more than "me too" lookalikes of current drugs. The FDA vets new drugs with reasonable care, but we now allow the creation of potentially dangerous new diagnoses without first having any careful and independent review. Changes in the diagnostic system should be subjected to a vetting process every bit as thorough and careful as for new drugs.

But who should do it? Probably a new structure within the Department of Health and Human Services that is broadly interdisciplinary—combining all the clinical professions with experts in public mental health, service delivery, health economics, forensics, and education. It could have a staff to conduct evidence-based reviews of the scientific literature—or perhaps better, should outsource such reviews to existing independent groups that will have no stake in the outcomes. Decisions should be based on open, explicit risk-benefit analyses that anticipate possible unintended consequences and also include impact on costs and allocation of resources. Consumers should be part of the vetting team. Everything should be posted in real time and completely transparent. New diagnoses should be subject to continued surveillance to ensure they are not being misused and do not have harmful unintended consequences.

Changes need to be gradual and incremental. It makes no sense to continue the practice of changing the entire diagnostic system at arbitrarily chosen intervals. Each diagnosis should be taken up individually in turns that are decided by the emergence of new research evidence. Change should not be just for the sake of change and must be supported by solid evidence and consensus approval. For the immediate future, changes in the diagnostic system will likely be determined much more by health services than by brain research. The neuroscience revolution is far sexier and more intellectually stimulating but, except for Alzheimer's, is very far from producing laboratory evidence to support diagnostic decisions.

Stepped Diagnosis: A Surefire Inflation Cure

We need to teach mental health clinicians and primary care physicians a completely different approach to psychiatric diagnosis. The current practice is to make a diagnosis on the first visit, based usually on very incomplete information obtained in a very brief interview with a patient who is going through one of the worst days of his life (and who may recently have been using substances that befuddle the clinical picture even more). The presentation on visit two is often quite different than it was on visit one. By visit five or six, things have usually stabilized and clarified enough so that an accurate diagnosis is a pretty good bet. Furthermore, many people naturally get better by then. The first visit is the worst time imaginable to make a definitive diagnosis, and diagnoses made in this way are often wrong.

So why do doctors routinely spring so prematurely? Why not watch, wait, learn more, see how things develop? Simple answer—insurance will often pay for a visit only if there is a *DSM* diagnosis generated during it. This is remarkably penny wise but pound foolish for the company—as well as being hazardous to the health of the patient. Once a definitive diagnosis is made, a definitive treatment is usually begun—and both are likely to be unneeded, harmful, and expensive. After all, people with milder problems have a fifty-fifty chance of being back to their usual selves within a few weeks without needing any diagnosis or treatment.

The best bet would be for insurance here to do what is done in many other countries—no diagnosis needed for the initial evaluation visits. This would save money and prevent mistakes. The second best and currently necessary solution—clinicians should underdiagnose and feel comfortable using "Not Otherwise Specified" categories that are less likely to carry stigma, to convey an aura of pseudoprecision, and to lead to unnecessary treatment.

Clinicians will need to be taught a new stepped approach to diagnosis that is the opposite of the "shoot from the hip" approach that insurance now requires and drug companies encourage. Definitive diagnosis should be made in the first session only in clear or urgent cases. For everyone else, the first several visits would be for fact finding, education, and to let nature take its course. Diagnosis would be made only after the dust has settled. This is the most direct and efficient way to stop diagnostic inflation in its tracks.[17]

STEPPED DIAGNOSIS

STEP 1—Gather baseline data.

STEP 2—Normalize problems: take them seriously, but reformulate positively as expectable responses to the inevitable stresses in life.

STEP 3—Watchful waiting: continued assessment with no pretense of a definitive diagnosis or active treatment.

STEP 4—Minimal interventions: education, books, computer-aided self-help therapy.

STEP 5—Brief counseling.

STEP 6—Definitive diagnosis and treatment.

Stepped diagnosis takes full advantage of the powerful healing effects of time, support, and placebos. In nonurgent situations, first-line diagnosis and treatment should be the least intensive, with a "step up" only when needed. Stepped diagnosis is cost-effective because it filters out situations where treatment will not be necessary and separates those who would benefit from psychiatric diagnosis from those who will do fine—or even better—on their own. It offers a tool for saving normality from psychiatry, and psychiatry from overdiagnosis and ridicule.

Taming Drumbeating

Every action has a reaction—diagnostic inflation and prescription drug abuse have gotten so far out of hand, and it is time for a pendulum swing toward better balance. There are three forces that together could powerfully push back against diagnostic inflation and possibly even reverse it. These are the professional organizations, the consumer advocacy groups, and the press. So far none has been sufficiently invested in diagnostic deflation, partly because each has been cleverly and systematically co-opted by the drug companies. In a fair and reasonable world, each would be on the front lines—fighting, not supporting, drug company marketing efforts. So far they have been on the wrong side of the line, but this could change rapidly, and they remain the hope of the future.

The medieval guilds were formed with two very different but compatible purposes in mind—to protect guild members from outside price competition and to protect buyers from poor quality products. Guilds were given a monopoly, but only on the condition they not abuse it and keep sacred the public trust. Modern mental health professional associations are guild derivatives but have broken the faith. They seem inclined to protect only their members and their staff bureaucracies, showing little regard for the preservation of quality or upholding the best interests of the public they are meant to serve. All of the mental health professional associations have remained remarkably passive in the face of massive drug overusage. None has raised much opposition to the recent false epidemics of childhood attention deficit disorder, autism, and bipolar disorder. Neutrality in these situations is not really neutral—it amounts to passive collaboration with bad diagnoses and inappropriate treatment.

It should be the ethical responsibility of professional associations to foster an open and informed public debate on mental health policy issues. The cynical view is that they fail to do so for reasons of self-

interest—i.e., going with the flow of ever-expanding diagnostic inflation brings in more patients to treat and the chance for drug company
subsidies. This may be part of it, but I think the problems go even
deeper and are harder to solve than simple financial conflict of interest. The professional associations are too selfish, yes, but even worse,
they are not very smart—as evidenced by the *DSM-5* debacle. Paro-
chial staff bureaucracies come to dominate their agendas, and they fail
to see beyond their own narrow interests. The associations are often
surprisingly ill informed about, and insensitive to, the patient care and
public policy issues related to diagnostic inflation.

Can this change? I think so. Exposure of their extensive ties to
drug companies has already forced medical associations to begin the
process of divesting relationships and regaining independence. If anything good can come from *DSM-5*, it will be increased awareness that
the highest loyalty of the guild has to be to the public, not to the guild
members. Failing to produce quality means losing your monopoly.
The American Psychiatric Association, having fumbled the diagnostic
inflation ball on *DSM-5*, will likely be more cautious about carrying
it in the future. It may even see the light and come finally to admit
that diagnosis has become too loose and drug prescribing too promiscuous. Organizations can change if their incentives are aligned with
public interest.

Consumer advocacy groups have done enormous good in furthering parity for mental health care, increasing funding for psychiatric
research, improving services, providing support, and reducing stigma.
Unfortunately, though, they have also become loyal but unwitting
(and more believable) lobbyists for drug company positions. This is
doubly problematic because they flunk the Caesar's wife test of being
above all reproach. Too much of their budgets are financed by drug
companies. In Europe, consumer advocacy opposes excessive medication use rather than enabling it.

There is also another, more subtle conflict of interest. Organizations always strive for more members. The larger the consumer advo-

cacy group, the stronger will be its political voice and financial clout. And the more people with the disorder, the less the stigma that attaches to it. Autism advocacy has done wonders, but a side effect is that perhaps half the people identified as autistic don't really have the diagnosis. As it matures, consumer advocacy will become more aware of the risks of overdiagnosis and will better balance the benefits of large membership rolls against the risk that some of those inappropriately included will in the long run be more harmed than benefited.

Investigative journalism is perhaps the best defense against drug company hype but has become something of a newsroom luxury. Reporters too often simply parrot drug company press releases without digging deeper into the always more complicated reality. Breathless stories promote the false conclusion that research advances justify the notion that all problems are brain diseases. Less attention is given to the fact that drug companies are much more engaged in, and better at, marketing and political lobbying than they are at scientific research. The industry pipeline of new drugs has been pretty empty for some time, but the flow of power in Washington and in state capitals never runs dry. When companies receive huge fines for criminal activities, it is usually back-page news or buried altogether.

There is some cause for hope. The media has definitely caught on to the dangers of psychiatric diagnosis, perhaps because *DSM-5* was so egregiously reckless and press insensitive. *DSM-5* coverage was well informed, extensive, worldwide, persistent, and often excoriating. Incredibly indifferent to external criticisms by professional groups, *DSM-5* finally did back down on many of its worst suggestions when these were scorched in the press. Big Pharma has also begun to take more hits as the impact of its excesses is increasingly felt by the most vulnerable—our kids,[18] the elderly,[19] the poor, and returning vets. The scandals of unchecked polypharmacy and iatrogenic overdose are also finally attracting the attention they deserve.

I would hope for a press that counters rather than echoes market forces, that monitors medical and pharmaceutical excess, and that finds a voice as public defender against diagnostic inflation and excessive treatment.[20]

Can We Deflate the Diagnostic Bubble?

Perhaps, but it won't be easy. Economic inflation is easy to start, but very difficult to stop. Sadly, the same is true of diagnostic inflation. The momentum behind it now seems irresistible. *DSM-5* threatens to turn inflation into hyperinflation. The drug companies will not easily surrender their strong monopoly stranglehold on a vulnerable and lucrative market. Politicians appear to be paralyzed by lobbying largesse, far from ready to enact appropriate external regulatory controls. Doctors prescribe reflexively. Patients accept claims gullibly. Professional associations either tacitly support or stand on the sidelines in the face of massive overusage of medication. Consumer groups have been co-opted.

Our diagnostic system needs to be protected from all the commercial and intellectual conflicts of interest—the publishing profits of APA, the drug company bottom line, the handouts given to professional associations and consumer groups, the eagerness of doctors to accept drug company perks, the love that experts feel for their pets. We need either to get the primary care doctors out of psychiatry or to teach them how to do it and give them sufficient time to do it properly.

The cures for inflation are simple and would be immediately effective if only we had the will to put them in place. But how to get the will, how to create the countermomentum. The *DSM-5* fiasco has had one positive impact—alerting the press and public to the importance of getting psychiatric diagnosis right and the dangers of getting it wrong. This should be the beginning of a thorough public and political debate on how best to reform our system of psychiatric diagnosis and to protect it from all the possible corrupting forces. Finding a better sponsor for *DSM-5* would be a great start. And the next obvious step would be to do what the rest of the world does—end direct-to-consumer advertising. Politicians won't care unless the public does. And the public won't care unless the media does. *DSM-5* would have been a lot worse but for media pressure, which finally brought the APA leadership partially to its senses. Let's hope the media are willing to take on Pharma and that public outrage and pressure results in sorely lacking political backbone. Diagnostic questions should be decided by what is best for the patient, not what is best for the doctor or the APA or Pharma or the consumer group.

We can do it. But will we?

CHAPTER 8

The Smart Consumer

Know thyself.
THE DELPHIC ORACLE

WHEN IT COMES to having a mental disorder, this is both the best of times and the worst of times. The best because there are so many effective treatments available and so many skilled clinicians. The worst because there is so much overtreatment of the people who don't need it and so much undertreatment of the people who do—and so many unskilled clinicians providing inaccurate diagnoses and inappropriate treatments. You can't trust our system for delivering mental health care to automatically work well for you, because it offers a crazy mix of good and bad options and is anything but a well-organized system. And curing diagnostic inflation through professional and regulatory changes will take some doing, won't happen quickly, and may never happen at all.

So where does this combination of opportunity and risk leave you? I would recommend having the skeptical "buyer beware" attitude assumed by all smart and well-informed consumers. You should give the same care to starting a treatment as you would to buying a car or a house or selecting your friends or a spouse. The decision whether or not to take a psychiatric pill or enter into a psychotherapy is often life changing. Never do it casually or passively.

Don't be daunted by having to play an important role in finding the treatment you need and avoiding the treatments you don't. You are used to making smart and tough consumer choices in all the other aspects of your life and this is really no different. The array of options for psychiatric diagnosis and treatment has proliferated along with all the other excessive consumer choices that characterize modern life. There are dozens of possibilities when you have to choose which camera, which TV, which shampoo, and especially which box of cereal among those aligned in that imposing wall at the supermarket. Having so many options is both good and bad—more choices, but also more chaff. I will offer tips on how to negotiate what might otherwise seem to be a confusing labyrinth of care (and noncare) options so that you can find what works for you.

Working with the Clinician

Psychiatric diagnosis requires a collaboration between you and your mental health clinician. He can't do it by himself. There are no objective laboratory tests in psychiatry, and therefore there is no way for anyone to diagnose your problems without your help. Here are things you can do to get the best result. First, be honest with yourself and with the clinician. It is no fun having to talk about psychiatric symptoms—particularly to a stranger. But accurate diagnosis is totally dependent on your complete openness and willingness to share your most embarrassing thoughts, feelings, and behaviors. However shameful or shocking your revelations may seem to you, be assured that they are part of the human condition and that the clinician will have heard similar (as well as much stranger and more embarrassing) descriptions numerous times before. It is the safest bet in the world that you are many times more judgmental of yourself than any clinician will ever be.

The key to psychiatric diagnosis is self-report, and this is impossible without careful and persistent self-observation. Start keeping a daily diary with a description of your symptoms as they arise. Note particularly the type of symptom, time of onset, severity, duration, level of functional impairment, stress, and the things in life that help you feel better or worse. Do your best to gather together as complete a record as possible of all past data that might inform your present diagnosis. It is especially important that you obtain copies of all your psychiatric and medical records. Until recently, it might have been difficult to gain access, but this is no longer the case. The records may sometimes be upsetting and/or inaccurate—so read them with strength and forbearance. Also know that if there are errors, you have the right to have them corrected. It is usually time-consuming and frustrating to get records, so having them ready well in advance gives you a head start.

When previous records are voluminous, it is helpful to maintain an updated chronological list of all the psychiatric medications you have ever taken—with dates, dosages, indications, response, and side effects. Also have a list of any other medications you are taking now or have taken in the past. Finally, maintain a chronological list of the names, telephone numbers, and e-mail addresses of all the mental health clinicians you have ever seen in the past and of any medical or psychiatric hospitalizations you have had. Keeping your own summaries helps to put things in perspective for you and ensures that important details won't be lost. It also saves valuable and expensive time so that you and your clinician can most efficiently focus on the meaning of what is happening, rather than recounting the blow-by-blow history of all the past events.

Neither you nor your current clinician should blindly follow the diagnostic impressions and treatment plans of past clinicians—these may have been wrong at the time they were made or have become dated by the things that have happened since. But, whatever its limitations, the past record almost always contains material that will shed illuminating light on the present situation. The time spent in collecting and updating your record will be richly rewarded.

Learn everything you can about the history of your problems, the most pertinent *DSM* criteria sets, and the most likely differential diagnoses. Occasionally a clinician may feel threatened or be defensive if you seem to know too much. But unless you are being obnoxious about it, this is probably a sign that you might be better off with a different clinician. The best single predictor of a good outcome of treatment is a good relationship. Liking your clinician and feeling she understands you and your problems doesn't guarantee she can help you, but it is a great start. If you don't feel comfortable with a clinician, find someone else you can communicate with. And remember that collaboration is always a two-way street—for you to get the best result, you have to really put your heart into it. It is difficult having a psychiatric problem, but it doesn't have to be tragic. People who take a matter-of-fact, information-seeking, businesslike, and collaborative approach to diagnosis and treatment planning usually wind up with the best outcomes.

How Can You Be Sure the Diagnosis Is Right?

Perhaps the easiest and least expensive way is to check out the diagnosis yourself. I used to recommend consulting the *DSM* criteria for assistance in this but have less faith in *DSM-5* because I think many of its suggestions will lead to overdiagnosis. The Internet has lots of good information, but many sites show clear signs of excessive diagnostic exuberance, often influenced by drug company marketing. There are many guides to psychiatric diagnosis for clinicians and patients that are more objective. I have written one myself that is meant to be a corrective to the excesses of *DSM-5*.[1]

The main things to check out are whether your symptoms closely fit the description of the disorder, have they lasted long enough to count, are they causing you considerable distress or impairment, and does it feel like they are just a temporary reaction to troubling events or are they more built in to your day-to-day life. You don't have to form an opinion on this right away. Keep a diary, chart the course, and see how things develop. If your symptoms get better on their own within a reasonable period of time, the questions will have answered themselves. But be sure to get help if they hang around, get worse, and continue to cause trouble.

Suppose your clinician comes up with a diagnosis that makes no sense to you given your own research. He could be wrong, especially if it was a snap diagnosis made after a brief interview. Or you could be missing something that he is picking up. When there are inconsistencies, don't be shy about politely asking the clinician to explain the rationale for her diagnosis and how she believes the criteria are met. Different clinicians often disagree on a diagnosis and it is often hard to tell who is right. Disagreement is particularly likely if you are young, your symptoms aren't classic, or if your problem is on the boundary with normality. It is always easier to call a strike when the ball is right down the middle of the plate than if it cuts the corner.

Whenever you are in doubt, get a second opinion from a different clinician, or a third or fourth opinion. And also see what your family thinks. Second opinions are particularly useful if your first treatment doesn't work and/or when there is any doubt at all about the diagnosis. My experience has been that some clinicians make the same diagnosis and offer the same treatment for almost every patient they see. Others develop an ephemeral enthusiasm for a particular diagnosis after attending a conference or meeting with a drug salesman. Too many clinicians go with the flow of the latest fad in diagnosis or the newest "wonder" drug that hits the market. You can be a useful restraining influence. And always expect your clinician to provide commonsense rationales and explanations for any diagnostic decision, and question them carefully if they do not. If the clinician doesn't have an open mind, if he gets mad, or if he can't explain the diagnosis in a way that makes sense to you, it may be a good idea to get another opinion.

Which Discipline Does Diagnosis Best?

This is a question I am often asked. Another variant: Is it important I see a psychiatrist for a diagnosis or can I trust my therapist? The answer is complex. No discipline has a monopoly on great diagnosticians or terrible ones. On average, the training and skill in diagnosis would roughly follow the hierarchy: (1) psychiatrists; (2) psychologists; (3) psychiatric nurse-practitioners; (4) social workers; (5) counselors; and (6) psychiatric occupational therapists. But many of the worst diagnosticians I have known have been psychiatrists, and some of the best have been nurses and social workers. So you can't go just by the diploma. There is more variability within professions than there is across professions. All the more reason to be a smart consumer, studying the issues on your own so that you (and your family) are in effect providing a well-informed second opinion and a monitor on the process.

It is especially hard to place primary care doctors in the hierarchy of diagnosticians. Some are absolutely brilliant at psychiatric diagnosis, but most lack the knowledge or are simply too busy or couldn't care less. This is important because primary care doctors are such heavy prescribers of psychiatric medicines. If your primary care doctor knows you well and has spent time with you before offering treatment, there is a reasonable chance it may make sense. But always be suspicious about a diagnosis and treatment plan when you are offered a prescription after a seven-minute visit or if the doctor offers to start you out with free samples. Nothing is ever free, and the doctor's decisions may have been too influenced by drug salesmen and by his desire to get you out of the office as quickly and conveniently as possible. Be aware that primary care doctors prescribe far too many medications in general and are particularly loose with antianxiety drugs (like Xanax) and antipsychotics (like Seroquel and Abilify). I would always get a second opinion before taking them.

I would recommend always seeing a psychiatrist if your psychiatric problems are severe and/or if you also have medical problems.

Is Psychiatric Diagnosis a Family Affair?

Almost always yes, but occasionally no. It is an inherent part of human nature to have biases and blind spots in the way we see everything. And the worst biases and biggest blind spots undoubtedly occur when we look in the mirror. Thus far we have described the uses of self-diagnosis, but we must also recognize its limitations and possible abuses.

Self-unawareness is the nature of the human beast, but it can be a special problem for people who have mental disorders. Severely impaired insight is an inherent feature of some psychiatric problems (e.g., schizophrenia, mania, delusional depression, anorexia, dementia, antisocial and narcissistic personality disorder). But insight can also be impaired in much more subtle ways in many of the less severe disorders. You may be the last to know that your depression (or anxiety or drinking) is causing significant impairment, and the last to want to get the help you need. Remember that two thirds of people with severe mental disorders fail to get the treatment that might make a huge difference in improving their lives.

This is where the family comes in. Loved ones can very usefully fill in gaps in information and insight and instill the sense of urgency that is often necessary before someone will seek help. They often provide a day-by-day awareness that might otherwise be lacking of the evolution of the symptoms and of their impact on functioning and on interpersonal relations. For this reason, I have always tried to include the family in every diagnostic evaluation of a new patient—whenever they are available and willing and if the patient is also willing. If geography makes personal interviewing difficult, phone contact or Skype is far better than nothing at all. Each family member can bring unique information and insights that in aggregate are much more likely to lead to an accurate diagnosis than would the conclusions of any one person. It is also useful if everyone in the family participates in monitoring the nature, course, and severity of symptoms, and if everyone is working from the same knowledge base in implementing the treatment.

There are two exceptions to this rule—situations in which active family involvement in diagnosis may not be a good idea and can cause its own set of problems. Most poignant is when the family is not loving and instead is working at cross-purposes. In the midst of a family feud, psychiatric labels can be used as dangerous weapons. This is particularly true when child rearing or custody issues are part of the dispute. The family needs to resolve the feud before they can be usefully involved in the diagnosis of any one of its members. Sometimes treating the individual successfully helps to reduce the conflict (which may have been triggered at least in part by that person's psychiatric problem). The family can then be brought together to play a constructive role.

There is a second exception. Young adults who are struggling to become more independent may need to sort things out for themselves without the involvement of their families. But these exceptions are rare. In most situations the family is a crucial ingredient in accurate diagnosis.

When Should a Psychiatric Diagnosis Be Reevaluated?

First impressions in psychiatric diagnosis, as in the rest of life, are not always accurate. Here are three situations when it is especially important to consider the initial psychiatric diagnosis to be no more than a tentative theory, not an established fact.

The first and most common is when the treatment plan that had been aimed specifically at that diagnosis has had unsatisfactory results after a fair trial (i.e., adequate dosing and duration). Treatment failure can, of course, occur even in the presence of a completely obvious and accurate diagnosis and an appropriate treatment. The first question should always be: Did you really take the medicine that was prescribed or do the psychotherapy homework that was assigned? A treatment shouldn't be judged a failure if it hasn't had a fair shot. But even good trials have on average about a one-third failure rate. This may call for a next trial of an alternative treatment for the same diagnosis. But another possibility should also always be entertained—that because the initial diagnosis was inaccurate or incomplete there was a less-than-optimal choice of treatment. Suboptimal diagnosis and treatment are always to be considered as possible causes of less-than-acceptable treatment response. A change in diagnosis and a new and more appropriate treatment sometimes work wonders.

Diagnostic failure is also often the result of missing the causative or complicating role of substance abuse (especially in younger patients) or of medical problems or medication side effects (especially in older patients). But missed or inaccurate diagnoses can and do occur for any number of other reasons—an incompetent diagnostician, a withholding patient, insufficient time for evaluation, or situations where diagnostic stability is low. Whenever the first treatment doesn't work well enough, it is useful to review how closely the diagnostic criteria have been met and whether something was missed during the first go-round. This should be done with your clinician—but it is also a good idea to check things out yourself and/or to get a second (or third) opinion.

Diagnoses made early in the onset of psychiatric symptoms are much less likely to be accurate and stable than those based on a longer track record. This is particularly true of diagnoses made of children (in whom developmental factors can lead to rapid changes) and of teenagers (in whom drugs, peer pressure, family issues, and problems in growing up can also play such a complicating role). Be tentative for all but the clearest presentations in young people. You can't always assume that a "lifetime diagnosis" (e.g., bipolar disorder or autism) will last a lifetime—especially when it has been based on incomplete information, a short course, and symptoms that occur early in someone's life.

The diagnostic process is a movie, not a snapshot. Making a diagnosis should never be static and frozen in time by a first impression. An initial diagnosis is just that—initial. It is a hypothesis to be tested and challenged by accumulating experience. Considering the course of the symptoms is a very important part of the diagnostic process, and the course is often revealed fully only with the passage of time. So keep an open mind and a watchful, introspective inner eye on the progression of symptoms and what it says about the diagnosis.

Some presentations of psychiatric symptoms seem to pop off the page of the *DSM* criteria set. These are classic textbook examples of the given diagnosis that no experienced clinician will miss and that you can probably make yourself. Some presentations are less obvious and will require considerable clinical skill to tease out. And there are some presentations that are, for the moment at least, so confusing that nobody, no matter how highly skilled as a diagnostician, can make them out. The more prototypical the symptom presentation, the greater (though never absolute) the confidence in the diagnosis and the proper treatment. The more muddled the presentation, the more tentative the diagnosis and individualized the treatment approach. Often only time will tell—the true nature of the disorder declares itself only as its course gradually unfolds.

The bottom line is to strive for diagnostic clarity, but not to impose it beyond what the available evidence allows. Changing a diagnosis midstream is often unsettling, but sticking with an inaccurate diagnosis is far more damaging. You and your clinician should feel comfortable testing the diagnosis with repeated systematic reevaluations. And when things are unclear, accept that they are unclear rather than jumping to a premature and inaccurate closure.

The Risks of Self-Diagnosis

The effort to become a well-informed consumer also has traps and carries risks. The most obvious is that the end result could be your becoming a badly misinformed consumer—leading to possible over-diagnosis, underdiagnosis, or misdiagnosis. It is always wise to stay skeptical about your self-diagnosis, to keep an open mind, and to check it out with family members and a mental health professional.

The most frequent cause of overdiagnosis is assuming that having one (or just a few) psychiatric symptoms means you have a full-blown psychiatric disorder. Many people have some symptoms some or all of the time—this is just part of life, not psychiatric disorder. Remember that you must have the full cluster of symptoms at a sufficient level of severity and duration before talking yourself into having a mental disorder.

The most common cause of underdiagnosis is insufficient infor-mation. This is also the most easily corrected. All you have to do is study more and be more thorough in your review of possible diag-noses. More difficult is the underdiagnosis caused by shame, denial, or your being an unusually stoic or hopeless sort of person. You will probably have trouble overcoming these on your own, so try to accept the help of loved ones and clinicians.

The most likely cause of misdiagnosis is to underestimate the role of alcohol and drugs in causing your symptoms. You may not have no-ticed the connection or you may feel the active urge to deny it because you don't want to face the thought of having to cut back. The second most common mistake leading to incorrect diagnosis is to miss the fact that your medical illness (or the medicine you are taking for it) may be causing your psychiatric symptoms. This is complicated and difficult to figure out on your own. Working it out will require the collaborative help of all of your medical and mental health clinicians.

The next risk of self-diagnosis is rare but potentially quite harm-ful. For some, the quest for information can feed a kind of emotional hypochondriasis. Try to remember that the individual symptoms of psychiatric disorder are extremely common and form an inescapable part of everyday life. Everyone has occasional flashes of anxiety, or depression, or attention deficit, or memory loss, or binge eating (and so on down a list of dozens of symptoms). But most people don't have a mental disorder. If you seem to have every disorder in the book, it is much more likely that you have none at all and are overreading the manual.

Finally, a little knowledge can be a dangerous thing. You may find sport in labeling not just yourself, but also your family, friends, and particularly your boss. This can lead to casting cheap shots, particularly in the heat of battle. Throwing diagnoses like darts can hurt the other person and cause you to experience a vicious cycle of blowback attacks. But for the vast majority of people, the benefits of self-diagnosis far outweigh the risks.

Beware Fad Diagnoses

If everyone suddenly seems to have a diagnosis or to be talking about one (be it ADHD, bipolar disorder, PTSD, or autism), assume it is being overdone and don't jump on the bandwagon. Also don't be overly influenced by your friends' diagnoses or media reports that a celebrity has a particular diagnosis or that a previously ignored diagnosis is now being discovered in lots of unsuspecting people. Cyclical diagnostic fashions come and go and leave much damage in their wake. Always be skeptical of the diagnosis du jour.

Beware the Drug Companies

The pharmaceutical industry will do its best to mislead you. It is in the business of making money by expanding markets and will do whatever it takes to recruit new customers. Drug companies are constantly being fined for unscrupulously passing out false information to consumers and to doctors, but they keep doing it because it is so profitable. Be particularly wary of drug company advertisements that are cleverly devised to move product by casting a wide diagnostic net, often catching people who don't need the product. Don't be trapped in it and don't let your children be trapped in it. Treat drug pitches with the same healthy skepticism you would have toward a glib used-car salesman. And don't assume that "Ask your doctor" will provide protection against snake oil. Your doctor may also be unduly influenced by the long and strong arm of drug company marketing. Beware doctors who have drug company logos on their pads, pens, and cups and are liberal with free samples. Be skeptical, but not cynical. Used correctly, medication can be very helpful and sometimes curative.

Herbal remedies that make mental health claims are even less regulated than drugs. Because they are not monitored by FDA, promoters of herbal remedies can and do make outrageous claims that are completely unsupported by evidence. There is no way of knowing whether their products are pure, safe, or effective. It is a fair assumption that all are a bogus rip-off.

The Internet is both the best and worst source of information on psychiatric diagnosis. Pick your sites carefully and with skepticism. Some sites are clearly drug company marketing tools; many others may be unduly influenced in less obvious ways by subtle and subliminal drug company marketing. Double- and triple-check things before believing them.

Natural Healing

Time and resilience are almost always on your side. Symptoms that are mild and stress related are probably just part of life and will get better on their own or if you make some simple life or psychological adjustments. I can't repeat enough times—don't jump to the conclusion that you are sick just because you are sad or anxious. Give yourself time to sort things out and to see how nature takes its course. And do the obviously helpful things that most people know they should do but don't. Exercise, exercise, and exercise—it is a great healer of both mental and physical problems. Make sure you are getting enough sleep—sleep deprivation causes psychiatric symptoms. Reduce or eliminate your intake of alcohol or drugs. Reach out to friends and family. Seek spiritual help. Figure out what you would most like to do and put more good minutes into your day. Identify which problems are causing you grief and then figure out solutions. Off-load whatever stress you can safely off-load. All this may seem trite and commonsensical, but trite, commonsensical solutions really do work for everyday problems.

Natural resilience and simple solutions won't work if your symptoms are severe and/or persistent. Real mental disorders need attention from a mental health clinician. Don't be shy about getting professional help when you need it, but avoid it when you don't.

CHAPTER 9

The Worst and the Best of Psychiatry

First do no harm.

HIPPOCRATES

AN ACCURATE DIAGNOSIS can save a life; an inaccurate diagnosis can wreck one. For many people, the day they are first diagnosed is a tipping point that will have a profound impact on how the future will unfold. It will be a terrific day if the diagnosis is done well and leads to an effective treatment. But done carelessly and callously, diagnosis can trigger an extended treatment nightmare. There is no better way to bring home the immense impact of diagnosis than through the life stories of people who have experienced it at its worst and at its best. First, we'll hear the harrowing accounts of eight resilient souls who suffered from incredibly incompetent diagnosis and crazy-making treatment. Their briefly told stories pack more impact than a mountain of dry statistics. Each has found a way out of the psychiatric labyrinth—but not without scars. Aside from all the practical problems, it is nightmarish having to face a distorting diagnostic mirror that reflects back someone strikingly different from who you are and who you want to be.

The clinicians in these sad stories (including me) ignored what should be the first and last dictum in medicine—First Do No Harm. It is painful to discover how many lives have been harmed and harmed badly when psychiatry is done badly. Psychiatric diagnosis at its worst leads to psychiatric treatment at its worst, and together the combination is a recipe for disaster. The casualties are a living and much-needed rebuke to the field and provide the inspiration and passion for the sizable antipsychiatry movement. Psychiatry must learn from its bad outcomes and take very seriously the often well-deserved attacks of its critics.

But in my view, monolithic opposition to psychiatry is far too undiscriminating in its broadside critique. Indeed, it seems to me equally impossible to be enthusiastically an uncritical psychiatric loyalist or a dedicated psychiatric debunker. Both positions miss the truth in their one-sided extremity. During my career in psychiatry, I have encountered many hundreds of patients who have undoubtedly been harmed by it. The beginnings of this experience thirty years ago had already inspired me to write a paper with the Hippocratic title: "No Treatment As the Treatment of Choice." Any responsible person must criticize psychiatry (and second others' criticism of it) whenever it is done badly and outside its proper sphere of competence.

But note this important disclaimer—the terrible diagnostic mistakes documented below do not in any way reflect the overall practice of psychiatry. You are about to read examples chosen because they illustrate the extreme of diagnostic incompetence and crazy treatment selection. The antipsychiatry movement, generalizing from worst cases like these, goes way overboard and condemns all of psychiatry. Their extremism would deprive those who really need treatment and can benefit greatly from it. The second half of this chapter illustrates the much happier outcomes achieved by most psychiatric patients.

For every patient harmed by psychiatry, I have known ten whose lives have been dramatically helped, in some cases probably saved. I recently experienced the odd coincidence of receiving two separate e-mails on the same morning each asking almost the very same question: How can I remain so high on psychiatry while at the same time being so critical of some of its recent trends and so fearful of the harmful impact of *DSM-5*? My answer came easily. Our field is blessed with powerfully effective treatments (the wide variety of psychotherapies and medications) allowing us to achieve excellent results—better than those in most of the rest of medicine. A majority of our patients receive substantial benefit; a substantial minority recovers completely; some are stalemated; only a few are made worse. As psychiatrists, we heal whenever we can, and we provide empathy and consolation whenever we can't. We are good at listening, caring, and using our experiences and personalities in the privileged journey helping others to heal, adapt, and help themselves.

Psychiatry done well is a joy forever—a useful and highly satisfying craft. Psychiatry done poorly is a dangerous form of quackery. Our field goes wrong whenever it overpromises, overtreats, and underdelivers. Not all of life's myriad problems are psychiatric illnesses. Not all psychiatric disorders are "chemical imbalance" or amenable to simply taking a pill. There is no shame in admitting that we still don't understand the causes of mental illness—the rest of medicine deals with much simpler organs, but the causes of most of the physical illnesses also remain obscure. Although we have general outlines that are valuable in guiding treatment, each person is unique and each treatment regimen must be something of a trial-and-error experiment to custom-fit the needs of that person. If patient and psychiatrist work and think hard and put their hearts into it, something good usually happens.

Mindy's Story: The Fad Overdiagnosis of Schizophrenia in the 1960s

We have two stories here. Story 1: A confused and rebellious teenager uses drugs, gets mislabeled as "schizophrenic," and is hospitalized for two awful years. Story 2: A young doctor participates in this overdiagnosis and damaging treatment and doesn't come to his senses until after she is discharged. Mindy Lewis is the girl. Once she got free of the repressive treatment system, she pulled herself together and matured into a wonderful woman and brilliant writer. Shame to say, I was the young doctor who helped make her life more difficult.

Mindy at fifteen had a striking physical appearance: her long, curly blond hair was everywhere, her smile mischievous, her eyes defiant, her demeanor provocative. Inside, though, "I was extremely anxious, self-conscious, self-critical. I thought of myself as bad, a failure, a nonperson and invented a persona who could be perceived as daring because inwardly I felt I didn't exist." Mindy was chronically truant from school, hanging out in Central Park with other kids who were abusing drugs. Her mother was unable to fathom how Mindy had morphed from her neat, well-behaved, ponytailed little girl into a scraggly, unkempt, pot-smoking insomniac, an alternately silent and foul-mouthed stranger who wandered barefoot around Greenwich Village. War escalated between them. "My mother was overpowering. She made it clear that there could be only one adult female in her realm."

Then things got really dangerous. "Coming home to an empty apartment after school, I'd sample the liquor cabinet, or inhale a cleaning-fluid-soaked rag. I passed out in stairwells where tough boys fed me barbiturates and forced their hands down my pants to 'revive' me, and for days afterward I was depressed and ashamed." Smoking pot added to her confusion: "My thoughts became animated in sensory synergy: I could see, hear, taste, and feel them. They weren't always pleasant. Often they accused: I was ugly, stupid, fearful, wishy-washy, a baby, a fraud, a nonperson."

Mindy started seeing a psychiatrist, but their discussions were going nowhere. "Finally, as if on a dare, I swallowed a handful of aspirin." Mindy's mother signed her over to state custody for admission to the celebrated long-term inpatient unit of the New York State Psychiatric Institute. This led to a prolonged treatment nightmare based on a profoundly wrongheaded diagnosis. The director of the hospital happened to be the famed cocreator of the term "pseudoneurotic schizophrenia." The idea was nutty on the face of it: you "uncover" someone's "inner schizophrenia," which could be identified even if there were no characteristic symptoms, simply because the patient was eccentric and the doctor was an "expert diagnostician" specially trained in the director's dower-stick method. The whole thing was phony but widely accepted throughout the country in the 1960s. I was a young and stupid doctor and bought into it.

Mindy was put through the horror show that passed for treatment in those days, and I was part of the team directing it. "Three times a day, we lined up for meds and I was given Thorazine, the standard drug for psychosis. If I tried hiding the pills in my cheek, the nurse would search my mouth and I'd be given a bitter-tasting liquid. Either way, the effect was the same: the drugs would nail you to the furniture, suck your life force, dry your mouth and fill your head with despair. Each time I swallowed the pills I wished the doctors could feel for themselves the deadening effects." The therapeutic environment was anything but therapeutic: "If you weren't depressed to begin with, this would do it: sitting around the ward smoking cigarettes, wearing hospital pajamas, unable to go outside, dulled by medication, getting fat on starchy hospital food and as a drug side effect. To break the monotony, we paced, played Ping-Pong, smuggled drugs, and unsnapped our pajamas for easy-access sexual exploration."

While we doctors thought we were "analyzing the transference" and providing the patients with brilliant insight and a "corrective emotional experience," Mindy saw it differently. "For the adolescent girls, going to a session was an occasion, like going on a date. I would leave open the top snap of my pajama top and dab on patchouli oil. I tried to impress him by being as freaky and interesting as possible. Illness was coin of the realm to get attention. Everything I did or said was labeled as a symptom; every passing mood was cause for alarm. I was actor and director of my own little drama. I tried to find the part of myself that knew I was OK, but my healthy self was a distant memory. Maybe the doctors were right and there was something irreparably wrong with me."

Mindy was saved by Mrs. Gould, the wonderful English teacher who ran the school and was one of the few sensible people working on the inpatient unit. "She saw me as a person, not as a patient. In her classroom we'd pull meaning from our shared experience of literature. But above all was her commitment to us, her 'brilliant children,' and her belief in our health, intelligence, and spirit. Although she never directly undermined the doctors, she was on our side when the rest of the staff didn't understand."

Mindy did luck out in her second doctor, "who was shy himself and talked about my painful self-consciousness with empathy and insight. Together we started working toward increased privileges. When I'd inevitably backslide and get into trouble, Dr. R. would fight for me to be given another chance. His trust in me worked, and gradually I was able to gain my privileges and get out of the hospital."

Overcoming setbacks, Mindy gradually forged a happy and successful life and a career as a graphic designer. Later she realized her ambition to be a writer and has published two books: *Life Inside: A Memoir* (published by Washington Square Press, 2003) and *Dirt: The Quirks, Habits, and Passions of Keeping House* (www.mindylewis.com). She now teaches writing workshops in New York City. Mindy doesn't have a schizophrenic bone in her body and never did. She has taught me two great lessons. First, she had the generosity of spirit to forgive my foolish collaboration in her psychiatric imprisonment. And second, she taught me always to look for what's fundamentally normal in people, not just what appears to be sick. We both, in our different ways, eventually succeeded in flying over the cuckoo's nest.

Todd's Story: The Fad Overdiagnosis of Autism Occurring Now

At fifteen months, Todd was happy and sociable, normal in every other way, but not yet speaking. His pediatrician overreacted and referred him for further evaluation. Big mistake. The testing found "profound" delays in both receptive and expressive language and introduced the possibility of autism or mental retardation. "How quickly we went from feeling that our son was a happy, normal child to being terrified of what was wrong."

By age two, Todd was speaking, but not yet using two-word sentences. Autism was the fad diagnosis of the day, and his pediatrician once again overreacted—now suggesting referral for a much more elaborate "Multidisciplinary Evaluation" at a very special center that was a three-hour drive away. Of note, Todd had moved up to speaking two-word sentences but, just to be on the safe side, his ever-conscientious parents chose to follow doctor's advice and keep the appointment. Another big mistake. Todd didn't sleep on the drive and his crankiness on arrival worsened when staff took away his favorite toy so "it wouldn't be a "distraction" and led him away crying for four hours of testing. He had never attended preschool and wasn't used to being apart from his parents. Todd returned tired, unhappy, and disengaged.

The testing results were devastating. Todd had profound delays in every area: speech, language, fine motor, cognitive, adaptive, and even gross motor (although he had crawled, walked, and climbed very early). His scores were below what he had done at fifteen months. The diagnosis—classic autism. The prognosis—grim. Todd might deteriorate further, lose the speech he had, never leave home, and never attend a regular school. It was suggested that his parents consider leaving their jobs to move Todd near to a specialized, intensive, forty-hour-a-week program costing around $75,000 a year. They received detailed instructions on how to apply for state coverage.

"I knew the scores and diagnosis couldn't possibly be right—they described a different child. The evaluators argued that they had many years of experience, were the experts, and that we were in denial. I pointed out that Todd showed much better skills at home, but was told that mastery means showing the skills in every environment. I didn't want denial to prevent my son from getting help, so I didn't dismiss the results—but I couldn't make sense of them because they didn't describe Todd."

Todd's parents are professors, so they started researching and discovered that young children should be tested in a comfortable situation, not when they are irritable, sleep deprived, and ripped away from parents. Within a few months, Todd was retested at a different center and scored normal for everything except receptive speech, which was borderline. Why the big difference? The new evaluations were much less stressful because his mother was present to reassure him. By age three, Todd tested normal in every area. At five, he has successfully attended regular preschool and passed his school district's evaluation with a comment that there is no reason he would have any difficulty in school.

How could the first set of experts get it so wrong? "I always thought it best to try therapy if there was a possible problem, but it can be very difficult to separate the evaluation process from the requirements for getting services. The evaluators who tested my son under such harsh conditions truly thought they were helping us and doing what was best for him; they wanted to make certain that he had as many services as possible in order to have the best chance of doing well. I wish that services depended on what each child needs, rather than on a misleading label and a standard set of recommendations. To do what was best for my son, we had to choose some services and turn down others."

Todd's parents had been misled and terrified by "experts" who were expert at pursuing autism at the slightest hint of his having any social or language difficulty. They got much better advice from another more trustworthy expert who understands the role of individual difference in development. "It is like dental work: it used to be fine to have somewhat imperfect teeth so long as they were healthy, but now they all have to be straight and perfectly white."

Having a diagnosis of autism, even briefly, has had negative effects persisting beyond the initial worries: "There are still people who make assumptions about my son and show lower expectations for him, surprised he can talk at all or is doing well in school. Some don't accept the second opinion and continually give advice as though he were dealing with challenges that he doesn't have (e.g., recommendations to start different therapies, special diets, special camps, to apply for grant programs for which he doesn't qualify, to obtain communicative devices that are unnecessary, to get therapy for nonexistent sensory problems, etc.). Even people who have heard the full story sometimes talk down to Todd, rather than understanding how well he can communicate with them. Other people reassure us that he will just be like scientists or engineers they have known. Comments like this make me wonder why it's necessary to give a diagnosis to people who are functioning well and are successful."

Susan's Story: The Fad Overdiagnosis of Adult Bipolar Disorder

Susan is thirty-one years old, happily married, the mother of two young boys, a middle school teacher who loves to hike, canoe, and ski. She was perfectly normal until her first child was born and is perfectly normal again now. "I always knew I would be a mother—I wanted children of my own and also to adopt. But I never expected motherhood to be as difficult for me as it was." Her first son, Eric, cried constantly and inconsolably for his first six months. Susan spent night and day trying to comfort him, but nothing worked. "I felt insecure as a mother. Here I thought I wanted all these kids, and I wasn't able to soothe the only one I had. I wasn't the capable, confident mother I thought I would be."

Finally, her pediatrician urged letting him "cry it out." After a harrowing week, this worked, and Eric began sleeping most of the night. But Susan stayed miserable and sleep-deprived: "I don't know if I had been holding myself together for my son, or if his wakings had damaged my sleep patterns, but I still couldn't get a decent night's rest. I felt completely burnt out." She did all the right sleep hygiene things—no caffeine, careful diet, exercise by day, relaxing sleep routine at night—but was still out of sync. Worried this was postpartum depression, Susan consulted a general practitioner who prescribed Prozac, Xanax, Ambien, and Lunesta—all within five weeks. The drug cocktail made things worse. "I remember crying and saying good-bye to Eric—not because I wanted to commit suicide, but because I thought I was dying."

Susan then asked to see a psychiatrist. "Near the session's end, Dr. A very nonchalantly said, 'I think you're a little bipolar.' I was shocked and started to cry. Dr. A explained her reasoning: I was worse on antidepressants, couldn't sleep, and had a slight family history of bipolar. She prescribed two atypical antipsychotics: Abilify and Seroquel."

Susan's family and friends couldn't believe the doctor's diagnosis. It went completely against their experience—there had never been anything the slightest bit bipolar about her. Susan read books and Web sites about bipolar disorder, and she too couldn't see herself in the descriptions. "The diagnosis didn't sit well with me, but I trusted my doctor."

She shouldn't have. The doctor surely meant well but was dead wrong—shooting from the hip she had missed the diagnostic target. Just as "schizophrenia" had been the fad diagnosis in the 1960s, bipolar disorder has recently exploded as the diagnosis du jour—pushed aggressively by misleading drug company marketing. Dr. A had fallen for it and was seeing a "little bit of bipolar" where in fact there was none. That's how fads work. Surely, Dr. A would have been more careful had she anticipated the enduring harm caused by her misdiagnosis.

The first casualty was Susan's self-esteem: "I had to wrestle with this new piece of my identity. I no longer felt normal. What crazy things have I been doing? People must have noticed, since it took Dr. A just a few minutes to pick up. I dreaded the day my son would find out. He deserved a better mom, a normal mom—one day he would realize that he wasn't normal either." And how could she get pregnant again— stopping her medicine might lead to recurrence of "bipolar disorder" and staying on it might hurt the baby.

Fortunately, Dr. A retired. The new psychiatrist was extremely skeptical about her diagnosis, remarking that Dr. A thought everyone was "a little bipolar." Susan was relieved of a psychic burden and was weaned off all the unnecessary medication. Soon she became pregnant again and delivered a baby son who was easy to care for. There was no return of postpartum depression.

Should be a happy ending, but it isn't. The bipolar diagnosis refuses to die, remains in her records, and still haunts Susan's life. First, it was the life insurance policy Susan wanted, to protect her children should something happen to her. She was rejected by four companies and discovered that bipolars are considered risky. Then she learned that she could not adopt a child. Susan and new spouse were ideal candidates— loving marriage, well educated, stable jobs, homeowners, highly motivated, stable, compassionate, and on and on. "Despite all things going for us, we found out we never had a chance because of my diagnosis."

Patient's rights regulations demand that inaccurate diagnoses be corrected, but the hospital has so far refused to admit the diagnostic mistake despite letters from other psychiatrists stating firmly that Susan is not bipolar. At least one cloud has lifted: "When my psychiatrist first told me that I am the best mom for my kids, I was speechless. I do have imperfections but feel thankful and proud to be the mother of my two little miracles. And I will keep fighting to get my records corrected."

There are many lessons here. Fads cause careless diagnosis. Clinicians should buck fads, not join them. Wrong diagnoses can do enduring harm that comes with no automatic expiration date. It is almost always better to underdiagnose than to overdiagnose. And doctors should never take at face value advice given to them by drug company sales representatives.

Liz's Story: The Fad Overdiagnosis of Childhood Bipolar Disorder and ADHD

Liz is twenty-three years old, a generally happy person now embarked on a life of public service, extensive travel, and loving relationships. "I have my ups and downs, like anybody else, but I don't think that makes me particularly crazy. Being able to say that and really believe it has been a long time coming."

Liz was a difficult child—hyperactive and prone to tantrums and power struggles. Neuropsychological testing at age five revealed high IQ—but the discrepancy between the verbal and performance scores was taken as evidence of attention deficit disorder and learning disability. Ritalin improved her handwriting but caused troubling side effects—a coughlike tic, compulsions, and depression.

"At age six, I would sometimes go in to the kitchen and hold a butcher's knife to my throat, not really thinking about actually killing myself but more just contemplating what would happen if I did. When I admitted this to my mother, she took me to Dr. Y, an expert on childhood behavioral and bipolar disorder at a famous medical school."

After a very brief visit, Dr. Y prescribed Zoloft. "What followed was a vicious cycle saga I still find infuriating and bizarre—it's unbelievable that a top psychiatrist put a young child through such traumatic and unnecessary experiences. The Ritalin meant to counteract ADHD caused depression, so they prescribed Zoloft, which made the ADHD worse. Instead of taking me off Zoloft or trying something else, my dose of Ritalin was increased, which caused worse depression, and so my dose of Zoloft was also raised."

This mindless chasing of side effects with ever-increasing doses of medication caused Liz's behavior to become increasingly erratic, uncontrollable, and wild. "I jumped out of the car as my mother pulled out of the driveway. I broke a glass and attempted to walk on the pieces. This was not me—I had never demonstrated such admittedly insane behaviors, neither before nor since. But I was just seven years old, and the high doses of two powerful drugs were just too much for me to handle."

On Dr. Y's advice, Liz was pulled from school and sent to a nightmarish day program. They responded to her drug-fueled defiant behaviors punitively, which made her more defiant. "My most vivid memories are of being dragged kicking and screaming into a small white locked room with padded walls. If I hadn't felt crazy before, that certainly did the trick."

After a few days, Liz's parents wisely rescued her from the program, stopped her medications, and returned her to school. Her behavior improved, but fights with parents over homework and discipline persisted and got worse as she began puberty. Dr. Y was again consulted— his national reputation overcoming doubts about the negative effects of his earlier interventions. The new diagnosis was childhood bipolar disorder, a concoction widely popularized by Dr. Y and his colleagues at the famous medical school. Liz's parents were told that antipsychotic drugs could help, and she was prescribed not just one, but two in combination. Her parents fortunately could not bring themselves to give her the drugs, and Liz refused to take any more medication.

"Although I continued to fight with my parents and teachers fairly regularly, I had my fair share of friends and got good grades. By the time I reached high school, I was a moody, angsty teenager, not unlike most high school students. I pushed myself to take honors classes and subsequently struggled with the unmanageable workload. My academic difficulties and the pressure I put on myself caused me to grow quite unhappy. After much debating, my mother convinced me to see Dr. Y once again."

This was another unfortunate triumph of misplaced faith over unhappy experience. Within minutes, Dr. Y was enthusiastically recommending two new medications. "I had been through too much trouble with medications and refused to take any more. After graduating from high school and leaving my parents' house, I have never since struggled in the ways I did before. My problems as a child would not have been so problematic if they didn't need things to be so structured and rigid— just the wrong fit for me. I don't doubt I have ADD but can live with it. The mental scars left by the doctors who tried to cure my growing pains with medication may never fully go away. They made me feel less than normal when I was young and still developing. Ironically, it is my very obstinacy, which they were trying to cure, that has allowed me to move past those experiences to lead a full and 'normal' life, whatever that means."

Brooks's Story: The Fad Overdiagnosis of Schizoaffective Disorder

In eleventh grade, Brooks had a six-month spell of sadness. After a few minutes of conversation with his family doctor, he was diagnosed as having "clinical depression" and medication was begun. "The impact of the label hit me like a ton of bricks. I developed a strong self-hatred for what felt like my puny, defective brain."

Eight months and numerous failed antidepressant trials later, Brooks experienced the added burden of a manic episode, probably triggered at least in part by the medication. "I felt I was here for a very special reason and I was going to do BIG things. When I was diagnosed with schizoaffective disorder, it was something I truly couldn't wrap my head around. The line between reality and fiction became quite blurry."

His hospital records state that Brooks had experienced delusional beliefs about decoding a message to save the planet and that he planned to write a book about healing to share with hospitals in the city. The delusional thoughts faded over the following year and doctors finally settled on the more accurate and much less stigmatizing diagnosis of bipolar disorder. But the psychological impact of the changing labels and constantly altered treatments was excruciating. "I believed I was wrong, period, and everyone else was right."

For several years, Brooks continued to feel severe dread, paralyzing anxiety, emotional pain, and a sense of being disconnected from friends and family. He worried that the numerous medications had permanently rearranged his brain chemicals, putting him on a crash course that could only get worse and worse. His dilemma forced a decision to either commit suicide or commit to fighting the battle wholeheartedly.

"There was an undying spark in the middle of my soul that said no. I was my own man and should decide for myself what's normal and what isn't. I refused to live without meaning." Brooks began an in-depth study of cognitive behavior therapy and created his own customized techniques for analyzing his emotional and cognitive states. He grouped these into what he calls "The Lens." "I knew there was something incredibly wrong in the metaphorical glass that was shaping my perspectives, beliefs, and emotional states, and I set out to correct the glass so I could see through it clearly and recover."

It worked. Using "The Lens" and other methods for the past twelve years, Brooks was able to define the life he wanted and feel well enough to go after it. He became a filmmaker, began to speak publicly about his experiences, and included many metaphors of his journey through psychosis in the first feature, *Kenneyville*. Brooks was also serious about that book he intended to write. Now entitled *The Lens*, it is nearing completion. "Of course there are life's ups and downs, but I've broken out of the intense fear, paranoia, sadness, and anxiety I once felt. I'm appreciative of everything in my life, including this journey. It has made me much stronger with a greater sense of connection to myself and others."

Bob and Sarah: Confusing Grief with Depression

Sarah's thirty-three-year-old son Bob committed suicide by taking a combination of antidepressants and sleep medications. The pills had been casually prescribed and carelessly monitored over a period of eight months by a doctor who saw Bob only a few times for a total of about thirty minutes and never once asked what was going on in his life. Bob had become disconsolate as he struggled through a painful and protracted divorce and difficult custody battle. He badly needed counseling help to deal with the emotional stresses and his practical problems, but this was never offered. All Bob got were increasing doses of unhelpful pills used in changing combinations—and these eventually became the vehicle he used to end his life.

Sarah had watched Bob's suffering evolve and had a premonition that things might end disastrously, but her many efforts to help were of no avail. She was understandably devastated: "I was numb, in a dream state, crying all the time, unable to sleep, eat, focus, work. I never realized how great my life was until I had no life. My family couldn't help—my father is a strong Catholic and withdrew from me; my sister started drinking again."

Two weeks passed with Sarah in deep, shocked mourning. Her friends suggested she go to the doctor, saying this would help her pain go away and get her going again. After a brief interview, he explained that she was clinically depressed and wrote a prescription for Lexapro, with a follow-up visit to occur thirty days later. "I told the doctor my son had taken Lexapro and had used them to kill himself and that I had anxiety about going on any medications because I saw how badly he had reacted to them. The doctor was clinical, brushing aside my fears and my loss. I needed someone who would understand and share the pain I was going through, not put a cold medical label on it."

Sarah took the pills for two weeks and got much worse. She became agitated and felt like killing herself to gain relief and to join Bob. The doctor incorrectly told her this couldn't possibly be a side effect of the medicine. "He said my suicidal feelings were all psychological and would go away if I continued the pills for at least thirty days. I stopped taking them immediately. This ended the suicidal thoughts, but not the suffering or longing for my son."

Sarah had to figure out on her own what she needed to do to go on living. "I began counseling, became active in grief groups, drew solace from devotion to my faith and church, practiced yoga, and threw myself into physical activity, into my work, and giving to others in my community. My son had a son, and I believe that Jason's love and needing me helped to save my life. I continue to live with my grief every day and always will, but at least I feel like living, and after two years, I can experience joy and laughter again."

Myra's Story: Prescription Medications Make Things Worse

Myra, a documentary filmmaker, was invited to an artists' workshop retreat where she met Jane, a writer. As they began talking about Jane's OCD, Myra worried she might have the same problem. "I was in talk therapy for depression with an experienced psychotherapist and had never taken any medication. But as Jane described her OCD, my ears perked up. That's me too! As a four-year-old, I had this habit of rocking myself to music to get to sleep, and it broadened into what seemed like a compulsion whenever I had a paper due, a new boyfriend, or some daunting task. And my thinking all the time about that dumb boyfriend seemed like an obsession. No doubt, I was OCD."

Myra sought consultation with Jane's psychiatrist, who fancied himself something of an OCD specialist and (mis)labeled many of his patients with it. Soon the diagnoses, the medications, and the side effects all started piling up in a mindless jumble. Dr. Z confidently confirmed Myra had OCD and also added that she might have traits of borderline personality disorder. He prescribed an antidepressant that helped her feel less depressed, but also made her jumpy, irritable, and hyperactive. To deal with this side effect, Dr. Z prescribed an antipsychotic that calmed her down but also knocked her out, made her drool, caused her to see double, and left her feeling like a zombie.

"I would tell my psychiatrist about all the side effects and he would always make a change. Ritalin to wake me up. Seroquel to put me asleep. Dial the Geodon down, maybe, or even increase it, telling me that ironically sometimes by increasing meds you circumvent their side effects. Maybe we should add on Abilify or Risperdal? Usually adding, rarely subtracting. All of these medications, and all of this strange reasoning, for the next few years. With my brain addled and spinning during that period, it was hard to keep track." As things got worse, Dr. Z decided that Myra had bipolar II and added on even more medication.

Myra's psychotherapist was skeptical. She saw no evidence of OCD or BPD or bipolar disorder. She was concerned that Dr. Z never asked for her insight into Myra's symptoms and background or returned her calls requesting his rationale for diagnoses that made no sense and medications that caused so many side effects and were making things much worse. "I knew I had to choose between my therapist and my psychiatrist. I felt like the child of divorcing parents—caught in the middle between two different theories of what was wrong with me. With the Celexa withdrawal and deepening depression, I felt like I had to grab at some kind of rope. I was in a dark tailspin, suicidal, unable to sleep at night, to stay up during the day. I couldn't stop thinking about all of the mistakes I had made in my life, all the opportunities to make different decisions, rerunning over and over again images of the past and bad memories in an endless film loop. I had no choice but to go with the psychiatrist."

Not a wise choice, but an understandable one. Myra was desperate for relief and Dr. Z always had a new suggestion—something to calm her down, something else to jump-start her. A constant chasing of side effects with medicines that caused even more side effects. Thankfully, the story has a happy ending. Myra went to a different psychiatrist who gradually withdrew her from the many medicines she was taking. She remains on only low doses of Lamictal and Wellbutrin, without side effects.

"I have no idea if they work at all but feel too scared to try life without them. Thankfully, with much less medicine, I've never hit a suicidal space again—just some brief depressions related to idle time from the usual pockets of unemployment that come with working in film and TV. I will never let anyone put me back on a crazy cocktail of drugs, and no one since Dr. Z has agreed with the 'OCD,' 'bipolar,' or 'borderline' diagnoses. Today I rely on exercise, friends, meditation, nutrition, and vitamins and would like to return to psychotherapy if I had more means and a steady schedule. I worry about professionals who call everything a disorder and prescribe unnecessary medications."

Through it all, Myra clung to work as a life raft, soldiered through the side effects, and has had great professional success. A grant allowed her to do a documentary selected for Sundance. She is now a sought-after filmmaker able to get regular work in a very competitive industry. And a much wiser consumer of psychiatric diagnoses and treatments.

Maria's Story: Missing the Drug Abuse

Maria had a challenging childhood with tempestuous parents. "My father was a driven man from humble beginnings with a short temper and little patience for 'emotional women.' Unfortunately, my mother was a very emotional and fragile woman with chronic depression." Both parents were frequently absent—her father on business, her mother with periodic breakdowns. His difficult character and her instability made for an impossible marriage. When Maria was eight, they divorced and fought a bitter custody battle that her father settled abruptly by taking Maria to live in another country. She didn't see her mother again for twenty years. A psychologist evaluating Maria for a custody hearing described her as well adjusted and loving despite all the troubles. Her father hired a series of nannies "who would end up pretty much raising me."

As a teenager, Maria experimented with drugs: first marijuana, then LSD and amphetamines. Her behavior became more erratic, and her performance at school deteriorated. "The drugs gave me the sense of belonging and respite from my tense home situation." After high school, she moved out, got a full-time job, and enrolled in community college.

"When I was twenty, I started having trouble sleeping and felt overwhelmed. I saw a general practitioner who diagnosed depression after a fifteen-minute visit. The diagnosis reaffirmed that there was something 'wrong' with me deep inside, but having a name for it reassured me it wasn't my fault." The doctor prescribed as carelessly as she diagnosed—no follow-up visits, just get in touch for refills. "The first day I took half a Paxil, it felt like methamphetamine. During class I could not stop my legs from shaking and had the almost uncontrollable urge to get up and run as fast as I could. I would wake with a start in the middle of the night, covered in sweat and fearing for my life. Seeking a 'calming' drug to counteract my agitation, I tried heroin for the first time—a plentiful drug in my circle of artists and musicians. My casual use escalated into a daily habit, and I was also abusing prescription medications whenever I could get my hands on them: Xanax, Klonopin, Valium, Vicodin, and Dilaudid."

Maria saw a psychologist who administered a series of tests to establish a diagnosis. "He said I was suffering from 'chronic depression' and 'generalized anxiety disorder.' Again, this validated me immensely. It was not my fault I was so screwed up! I did not question how my drug use or even the unresolved (and very real) issues in my life could have affected the results of my tests." She was referred to a psychopharmacologist. "Our visits lasted roughly ten minutes. He kept giving me more meds. As a drug user, I was ecstatic that now I had a prescription for a drug I had been taking recreationally. But things in my life got worse."

No one identified Maria's drug use as the basic problem, and no one made any attempt to help her stop it. Instead they just kept piling on new diagnoses and throwing new drugs into the confused mix. When she didn't respond to one pill solution, her diagnosis would be switched, and a different one would be tried. Soon she was pronounced bipolar and even more medication was prescribed. "I was taking a mixture of many illicit and legally prescribed drugs and began to feel very depressed. I had a hard time getting up in the morning, quit school, and for the first time since I was fourteen, did not have a job. I no longer answered my phone, my shades were always drawn, and my days consisted of leaving the house only to buy drugs and sitting around watching TV. I was in full, addictive mode, seeking meds by manipulating my psychopharmacologist—especially the Klonopin, which had a pleasant and immediate effect of relaxation. If I mentioned trouble sleeping I could always get him to prescribe more 'fun' drugs."

Who needs a drug dealer if you have an overly compliant doctor who is no more than a pill pusher? Maria was hooked: "If I feel this bad *on* medication, how bad would I feel if I stopped it? My life became increasingly chaotic and unproductive. I lost hope."

Nothing was working, and Maria's psychiatrist recommended she be placed in a closed psychiatric facility. He told her father that Maria's condition was genetic and permanent, would always require intensive medical care and medication, and that he should "let her go." A different consulting psychiatrist confirmed her previous diagnoses and managed to add three more—obsessive-compulsive disorder, borderline and passive aggressive personality disorders. "I was twenty-four years old, had at least eight diagnoses, was taking fifteen pills a day, and seemed like a totally hopeless case."

Luckily Maria's father, a successful businessman expert at finding solutions to difficult problems, would not accept doctors telling him there were no solutions. He arranged for Maria to enter a long-term therapeutic community specializing in addictions. "I was sure of two things—that I would need to continue medication and that I would be out of the facility in a couple of months."

Both predictions were wrong. Maria stopped using street drugs, gradually weaned herself off prescription drugs, and stuck with the program. She couldn't believe how good she felt. "How strange that I could be normal. Difficult and happy periods come and go, just as they do in everyone's life. But I learned to accept them as part of life. Twelve years have passed, and I am now thirty-seven, with a rewarding job and a wonderful man at my side. It often occurs to me: What if my father had given up, had listened to the professionals? Where would I be? I also think I am lucky that the mix of prescribed and illicit drugs did not kill me. Contrary to what I had always believed, contrary to what psychiatrists told me, I was normal when I got off the drugs from the street and the ones they had prescribed for me."

Balancing the Bad with the Good

Wherever the art of medicine is loved, there is also a love of humanity. Cure sometimes, treat often, comfort always.
HIPPOCRATES

The next part of this chapter is devoted to providing just a few commonplace illustrations of the day-to-day successes of psychiatry—a much-needed balance to put its occasional failures and mischiefs into proper context.

Roberta's Story: Pets Kept Her Alive; Pills Cured Her Depression

Roberta is a fifty-eight-year-old high school English teacher who laughingly describes herself as "a spinster, a crone, and a hag in the very best sense of each of these words." But she is not alone in life. She has many good friends, lives in the cherished home where she was born, and is surrounded by beloved pets—a pig, three dogs, four cats, an iguana, eight chickens, and twelve songbirds. Her father died suddenly when she was only eight and her mother three years ago after a long illness that required much care giving. Roberta had always handled all of life's stresses with great grace and infectious good humor.

Roberta's psychiatric problems came as a complete surprise and began when her brother sold off her mother's jewelry and treasured antiques to buy himself a boat—doing this without consultation, without permission, and without apology. She couldn't forgive him or forget the blow to their relationship. Her brother had been her best friend and was her only remaining family member. "I felt alone—and now understood why Dante reserved his lowest circle of Hell for those who betray a trust. I was stunned and spiraled downward into deep depression."

Roberta cried constantly and couldn't eat, sleep, concentrate, speak to friends, or smile. Getting out of bed was a struggle. Each day at school felt like torture and lasted for an eternity. She was agitated, with an "awful pit-of-the-stomach feeling" that ruined her waking hours and churned her through fitful sleep. "The deeper I sank, the more I wanted to die. One day I was at the laundry and I crawled on the floor, praying for death. It is said that there are no atheists in foxholes. Perhaps the same could be said of the deeply depressed. At home I would pace the floor."

Roberta met with a sympathetic therapist who correctly diagnosed depression. "But she didn't seem to understand the depth of my pain. I needed someone who was willing to do something for me *now*! Not just talk." Then things got dangerous. "By this time I was ready to commit suicide. I would get through the day only by telling myself I could always go home after work and take all my heart medicine in an overdose. This gave me a feeling of peace—I could end this misery whenever I needed to. The only thing that kept me alive was holding my pets and that I couldn't bear the thought of leaving them behind. Life or death was a day-to-day decision. Friends rallied around and gave me support in wonderful ways. Even so, the depression and feeling of isolation continued and got even worse. I thought I would never get better."

Roberta's story has a happy ending. A friend who also had depressions convinced her to go to a doctor. "She prescribed an antidepressant and said it would take weeks to feel a difference, but assured me that I would get better." Eight weeks, four doctor visits, and three increases in dosage later, Roberta actually did begin to feel better and soon recovered completely. "One day at a school meeting, I made a smart-ass remark to a friend sitting next to me, and she said, 'You're back!' I was. I could laugh and smile again. My appetite for food and life returned, and I stopped having that sinking feeling in my stomach. I was able to look at things more objectively and to make plans for the future. Looking back, the combination of my pets, loving friends, and medication brought me back to normalcy. I have my life back and I am so thankful. Now my fear is that someday, for some reason, the depression will return. I want never to feel that again. At least this time I will know what to do about it."

Bill's Story: Keeping Mood Swings Under Control

Bill's bipolar disorder has not prevented him from having a wonderful thirty-five-year career as city planner. At twenty-nine, Bill was on top of the world, serving as project manager for a major urban renewal project—a highly stressful but "dream" job. Then the bottom fell out—the funding was pulled, the job was lost, and "my hypomanic energies turned into depression." He was successfully treated with medicine and psychotherapy, a new job came along, and everything went well for six years, during which he needed no medication.

Bill's second depression hit out of the blue and was much more dangerous. "I dragged myself to work but felt listless, hopeless, distractible, and severely suicidal. I was referred for hospitalization and ECT, but luckily the antidepressant medicine kicked in just in time and the depression lifted. Then I went overboard in the other direction with full-blown mania—racing thoughts, grandiose plans for multiple impossible projects, and strange ideas. I thought everyone was watching me and reporting to the police or FBI. And I did strange things—like buying thirty huge books on the universe and the history of mankind without thinking about the fact that they were far too heavy to carry home and far too long for me ever to read. Fortunately, lithium worked, and soon I was back on even keel."

Bill stayed stable for the next fifteen years until he, his wife, and doctor all agreed it was worth a try going off lithium because of the long period without episodes and the fact that the medicine seemed to dampen his personality. The trial failed. "Within three months, I was hypomanic again and realized I'd always need medicine. So we switched to another mood stabilizer, which has worked like a charm for the last seventeen years. I believe I will always be vulnerable, but the medicine gives me stability."

Bill retired from city planning at sixty-five to begin a second career. "And now I am a psychotherapist in training with fifteen patients, most of whom are doing well in treatment with me."

Susan's Story: Controlling Panic Disorder and Agoraphobia

Susan is a thirty-five-year-old caretaker, volunteer, writer, and self-described collector of college degrees. At age twenty, she was a college student looking forward to a bright future, a social butterfly with many friends. Then suddenly without warning, rhyme, or reason, Susan's life turned into a living hell filled with panic attacks and constrained by the urgent need to avoid anything that might provoke them.

"The first one came out of nowhere. I planned to meet friends for a movie and started having strange thoughts of getting sick in the theater, or going nuts in front of everyone. I couldn't breathe, my chest was pounding, and I felt terribly dizzy. I had no idea what was happening and felt terrified I was going crazy."

Attacks gradually became more frequent, occurring whenever Susan tried going out to a movie, dinner, or party—any social event or place that she couldn't escape if she felt panicked. "Slowly the list of things I avoided grew longer and longer until I was a total homebody, leaving my apartment only when absolutely necessary, and only with a friend. I wanted more than anything to die."

After eight years, twenty-one primary care doctors, dozens of medications, and far too many MRIs and other tests, Susan still had no answers. Medical doctors frequently miss the diagnosis of panic disorder because they don't know that its physical symptoms are caused by hyperventilation. This leads to unnecessary testing and aggressive treatment of imaginary medical problems.

At wit's end, Susan finally saw a psychiatrist, Dr. S. An hour later, she had clear answers to what caused her physical symptoms and could control them by slowing down her breathing. Her world brightened when Dr. S. confidently said she would definitely get better. He was right. Susan used her treatment to gradually face down her fears and regain her life. "Now I go out with friends, shop at the mall, go to the cinema, use public transportation, and do anything I want on my own. I continue to improve and set realistic goals each year. Flare-ups of agoraphobia come back when stress gets high, but because I am aware of what is going on, they are short and I know how to fight through them to stop avoiding. I love my life and want to share what I went through with others to help them not suffer needlessly the way I did."

Paul and Janet: Facing Down PTSD

The car spun out of control and crashed into a tree—instantly killing Max, age fifteen. The family tragedy happened on a slick and curvy road during a ski trip to Switzerland. Max had occupied the vulnerable front seat because he was most liable to get carsick. His parents and sister Annie were all badly injured but survived and rehabilitated physically within a few months.

Paul and Janet never talked about the accident, but they never recovered emotionally from it. Max's room was left as a shrine to his death in the same chaotic mess that always characterized his life—not a paper moved, not a shoe or baseball cap put in place, his last half-completed homework just where he had left it. He was constantly in their thoughts, but neither dared speak of him or cry or share their suffering openly for fear of upsetting the other. "We were both in suspended animation. Going through the motions of life, but numb and not really living. We grew apart, blaming ourselves, blaming each other. Neither of us had much to give Annie—our hearts were broken, our brains in turmoil, our tanks were empty."

Both parents were outwardly stoical, inwardly seething with nightmares and haunted with constant daytime images of Max's limp and mangled body. Paul could no longer drive a car for fear he would lose control of it again and kill someone else. Car trips were avoided by both parents whenever possible or were endured with dread. A year after the event, they still startled at the sound of a car horn, or skid, or acceleration. Neither could concentrate, or eat, or sleep well; both were irritable, living under a cloud, walking on eggshells.

Annie was subdued and intermittently tearful, but far less psychologically damaged than her parents. She missed her brother and felt very sorry for him and for her parents, but she had no memory of the crash and was better able to go back to her previous life of school and friends. For Paul and Janet: "Our lives stopped when Max's life stopped. It should have been us, not him. He had everything to look forward to. We have nothing to live for. What a criminally stupid idea to go on a ski trip and to drive on unfamiliar roads."

Paul is a cardiologist, Janet an OR nurse. It was four months before he was physically and emotionally ready to return to work; three months for Janet. Work was a salvation for both—the only place where they could function near normally. But Janet had panic attacks when dealing with trauma cases and had to restrict herself to elective surgery. And Paul felt unable to treat teenagers.

"Neither of us wanted psychiatric help, but we both knew we needed it. Our family doctor did his best, but the antidepressants and sleeping pills didn't help. The psychiatrist said we would never get over the pain of losing Max, but that we could and had to find a way forward—that we owed it to Annie, to the memory of Max, and to each other to make the great sacrifices treatment would require. We would have to face fully and share the pain of losing Max—no more suppression of feelings or secret grieving. That meant going over our memories of him together and finally accepting his death by clearing out his room. We came to understand that we could be true to the memory of Max without trying to stop the clock or pretend he wasn't dead. We would also have to face, not avoid, the horror of the accident. That meant discussing it, looking at the horrible pictures, beginning to drive again. The treatment was a wrenching, dreadful experience, but it did give us back not all, but part of ourselves and our lives and freed us up to love each other again and to be parents to Annie."

There is no pill for grief, and the medications for PTSD are not very effective and sometimes add new problems. Everyone has a personal way of grieving and dealing with catastrophic life experiences. For many, the best approach in the long run is the most painful in the short. Acceptance and catharsis require the reliving and sharing of the horrible memories and the gut-wrenching feelings. Facing the event rather than avoiding it is often the only way of gaining a measure of control and peace of mind. This can be done with family and friends, but if the feelings are tightly sealed, then a therapist is helpful, sometimes essential.

Peter's Story: Beating the Family Curse of Melancholia and Suicide

It looked like Peter had somehow defied the odds. Despite a strong history of depression and several suicides on both sides of his family, he had happily sailed through a charmed life, succeeding brilliantly at everything. At age forty-six, he ran a large business, had a lovely and happy family, and was a pillar of his church and community. Then, after a relatively trivial business reversal, things quickly began to fall apart.

"I don't know why, but I gradually lost all confidence in myself and in my ability to make the right decisions in business and with my family. I started ruminating about all the mistakes I had ever made in my life and felt that I was letting everyone down at work and at home. I blew up little worries all out of proportion and couldn't sleep because my mind was churning with catastrophic scenarios of future failures. I lost fifteen pounds and felt agitated and frozen at the same time."

Peter's brother, a physician, suggested he get a thorough medical workup and also consult a psychiatrist. Peter was fine with the workup but opposed to the psychiatrist. He was an independent and private person and was fearful he might be succumbing to the illness that had caused so much suffering to his family. Instead he hoped to ride out the storm and pull himself and his business affairs together on his own.

All the medical tests came back negative, but Peter's symptoms worsened. "I became completely irrational about money—convinced I was driving myself and the business into bankruptcy, even though my wife and accountant both kept showing me healthy balance sheets. I insisted that the IRS would audit us and that I would wind up going to jail. I began to feel hopeless and suicidal—if I had had the energy and the means, I probably would have killed myself. The pain was that bad, and I couldn't get over the crazy conviction I had done something criminal and had to be punished for it. I didn't want to be a burden on my family and put them through my public humiliation. It was all completely nuts, but I believed it."

The family gathered together and prevailed on Peter to see a psychiatrist. After hearing him out, the psychiatrist advised Peter that he was right to think the diagnosis was depression, but wrong to think the prognosis was bleak. It might take time, but the treatment would almost certainly work if Peter would suspend disbelief and really put his heart and his hopes into it. The first step would be medication, to be augmented next with cognitive therapy as soon as Peter began to feel up to it. Suicide as an option had to be taken off the table—it would create a much worse burden on the family and made no sense when the odds for recovery were so favorable.

"What a relief. We really hit it off on a personal level, and I felt hopeful again for the first time in months. It took me a while to really come out of the depression, but I never hit bottom again and was able to treat my worst fears as fears, not realities. It has been three years now and I haven't had a relapse. I will never feel completely safe about having another serious depression, but at least I can catch it sooner and get it fixed."

Cleo's Story: Focusing in on ADHD

As a girl, Cleo talked so much people would joke that she had swallowed a radio, and she was so active she often bruised herself in falls or by banging into walls. At school, she rocked in her chair and had trouble following her teacher but still managed to be the best student in the class.

Cleo's parents were both professors of Lebanese background who had migrated to Australia when she was an infant. They felt overwhelmed by their daughter, hired a nanny whose sole job was containing her, and decided not to have any more children. "I didn't get diagnosed because my parents had a cultural bias against accepting mental illness and the school was satisfied, since I was doing so well academically. Also they didn't know what a normal Arab was like, let alone an abnormal one."

Things deteriorated when Cleo was fifteen. She became depressed, doubted herself, feared failure, felt cut off from family, was without friends, and had suicidal thoughts. "My parents again rejected the notion of mental illness, so I had to deal with mine alone. Being sheltered made me unprepared and vulnerable for a world that seemed so cruel. Even seeing happy people made me burst into tears, I so desperately wanted to be like them."

Despite her inner turmoil, Cleo graduated from high school six months early and began college—majoring in psychology because she hoped to understand herself better and help others. But, at seventeen, she wasn't ready. "Gone were my A's! Everything was so much harder. For the first time in my life I was a C student, distracted by the simplest things, and my mind kept hopping from one thought to another. I'd start writing notes, then realize the lecturer had changed slides, my sentence was incomplete, and I had forgotten what he'd just said. I could barely read a page before I lost track of what I was reading and had to put a ruler under each line because I kept losing my place. Other thoughts would pop into my head and I kept getting up to do other things, then remembered I was supposed to be reading. No matter how hard I tried, I could not achieve the grades I was used to. I felt like a failure."

Cleo was referred for treatment but didn't like her therapist. "I found the lack of clarity in my diagnosis or discussion about it unacceptable and frustrating. I could not make sense of the chaos that was created by my disorder. I felt that to treat my illness, I'd have to know what it was."

Cleo got a second opinion and the new therapist explained ADHD and how it was impacting her life. "Receiving a definitive diagnosis gave me a huge sense of relief, and I felt I was finally understood. I also realized I was not a freak, that there were others like me, and that it was not my fault that some things about me irritated others. My therapist helped me understand what it means to have ADHD and introduced me to many strategies and study techniques. He lent me books on ADHD and referred me to many useful Web sites. I began to educate myself, researched my disorder, and became more aware of my symptoms and how to deal with them."

Cleo improved greatly and graduated from college. But she still had considerable difficulty concentrating and began taking Ritalin to help with it. "The results were astounding. My attention span and focus were dramatically increased, and I found myself being able to sit down and type at a computer for three hours." Cleo successfully completed her degree with first-class honors. "After a decade of experiencing a disparity between my actual abilities and my academic grades, I finally felt like I was meeting my potential. I finally felt like myself again. The combination of medication and psychotherapy worked perfectly for me. Receiving the correct diagnosis has helped me deal with my distress, take responsibility, and feel in control of my life." Cleo is now an educational psychologist helping others meet their potential.

Henry's Story: Living with Schizophrenia

Henry was a shy and introverted child who grew up to be a decidedly peculiar teenager obsessed by spiritualism, science fiction, and conspiracy theories. By age eighteen, Henry had elaborated the unshakable conviction that he could communicate with the souls of his dead ancestors by receiving their voice commands and decoding special messages from them on the Internet. He believed he had been given the special assignment of protecting the United States from the dilution of its Caucasian stock and the hostile takeover by a foreign power or the United Nations. Henry was fearful, hypervigilant, and could not ever let down his guard. His enemies had gained control of many government agencies, acquiring technology that allowed them to observe his movements, monitor his thoughts, and exert control over his actions.

Henry slept by day, read conspiracy literature and searched the Internet by night. He dropped out of school, increasingly withdrew from the real world, and remained in more or less constant contact with his voices and in thrall to his delusions. His parents shared Henry's general political orientation but were alarmed by his increasingly extreme and bizarre thoughts and behavior. They felt paralyzed. "Henry was retreating into another world we couldn't enter. He would become very angry and shout us down when we tried to talk to him or get him to do anything. He refused to go to the doctor, and we were really afraid of him. We got rid of our guns because we were worried he might become violent."

The crisis came when Henry's mother tried to clean his room because she felt it had become a health and fire hazard. Henry took this as a hostile act and assumed she was now acting under orders from the enemy. He pushed her out the door violently and threatened her with a knife—but then felt terribly guilty, began crying uncontrollably, and shouted his intention to kill himself.

An ambulance was called, and Henry was admitted to a psychiatric hospital. The diagnosis was schizophrenia and he was started on an antipsychotic. The medicine worked well, and Henry calmed down quickly. But recovering reality has been a much slower process that is not complete five years later. "I still have the voices, especially when I am stressed or have nothing to do. But I can usually tell they aren't real. It is a big relief not feeling watched and controlled all the time, but I get sad sometimes that I don't really have a special mission to save my country. It is a letdown not having a clear purpose anymore. I am trying to find other things to do and ways of keeping busy."

Henry was able to develop a trusting relationship with his psychiatrist. The treatment combines medication with weekly psychotherapy focused on reality testing and social skills training. Henry graduated from high school, has had only one additional brief hospitalization, and works very hard at therapy and at making a good life for himself. He turned his abiding interest in science fiction to great advantage, earning money buying and selling memorabilia on the Internet and making friends at science fiction conventions. Recently he began dating a girl who is also a science fiction fan.

Brandy's Story: Getting off the Roller Coaster of Border-line Personality Disorder

Brandy was an emotionally intense, impulsive, and self-destructive young woman who led a troubled and tumultuous life. She never had the slightest difficulty getting into relationships but was consistently unable to end them without feeling furious and deeply hurt. The same pattern recurred over and over again. Brandy expected too much, would get too close too soon, become fearful of rejection, and act in an angrily manipulative way that guaranteed that her worst fears would be realized. "Then when I was abandoned, I couldn't control myself and did really stupid things. Losing a boyfriend made me feel like I was being torn apart inside a black hole. Cutting myself calmed me down—physical pain beats emotional pain any day."

Brandy's school, family, and social life were almost as erratic as her love life. She is really smart but couldn't stick to the task at hand and was always disappointing and disappointed. At twenty-five, she was thirty credits short of graduation after attending four different colleges and having dustups at each. Except for one sister, Brandy was not on speaking terms with her family, and her friendships usually lasted only months before ending stormily. Therapy hadn't been the least bit helpful—many promising beginnings that all ended badly.

Things hit bottom when Brandy made an impulsive suicide attempt, taking ten sleeping pills. She was admitted to the hospital overnight and referred to an outpatient program that specializes in dialectic behavior therapy. "I felt different about DBT from minute one. The people understood and accepted me but also expected me to change and to take more responsibility for myself and my actions. I couldn't manipulate or fool them, but I felt they really cared and knew how to help me help myself. I like my therapist and want to be more like her."

Brandy was taught concrete ways of reducing her self-destructiveness. She flicked rubber bands on her wrists instead of cutting them with a razor.

She practiced going slow at the start of relationships, having fewer expectations during them, and ending them on a calm note. Brandy finished college and is now working on a master's degree in counseling. "I still have a temper and can be fragile, but I am maturing fast and think I am almost ready to use my experiences to help other people."

Adam's Story: Overcoming Obsessive-Compulsive Disorder

Adam was the perpetual ABD—an "all-but-dissertation" PhD candidate who had been working on his research project for seven years and seemed incapable of ever completing it. Each time his adviser said that it was ready for submission, Adam would become obsessed with what to him seemed its glaring imperfections and was always convinced it needed a lot of reordering and cleaning up. He would churn all night with anxious thoughts of failure that were neutralized only when he began an extensive revision—adding new material, scrapping chapters and references, adding new ones—essentially guaranteeing that he could never wind up the work and have to hand it in for review.

"I knew it was crazy and counterproductive to keep redoing my dissertation, but I felt stuck and like I had no control over the process. Constantly revising was stupid, but I got too anxious if I didn't. And it wasn't just the dissertation. I had to spend an hour every day getting myself dressed—following a complicated ritual that had to be repeated perfectly from start to finish if I didn't get each and every step just right. My day was also filled with dumb eating and sleep rituals, and I had to spend a lot of time praying."

Adam's rituals had begun in childhood and had gradually accumulated throughout his life so that they increasingly occupied almost all of his time. All along he had resisted treatment—fearing it would make him even more anxious by interfering with his rituals. But he finally reached the point of no return when his dissertation adviser threatened to drop him from the PhD program if he didn't meet the next deadline for submission.

"The psychiatrist was a good guy and understood the pressures I was under. He explained that the only way to beat OCD is to face the anxiety, not neutralize it with rituals. Getting my PhD was simple but scary—I just had to hand in the latest draft of my dissertation without rereading a page of it. He helped teach me techniques for dealing with the anxiety. I really had no choice and took the plunge. It was a terrifying few weeks, but the committee quickly approved my PhD and I was on my way."

Adam's many other rituals proved more intransigent because they were so built into his daily life and were less obviously destructive. But two years of therapy and medication gradually gave him his day back. "I still have a few pet rituals, but they don't take up much time and I feel like a free man for the first time on years."

Getting It Right

Done poorly, psychiatric diagnosis can be an unmitigated disaster leading to aggressive treatments with horrible complications and life-shattering impact. Some of the worst mistakes are made by clinicians who combine ignorance with arrogance—who don't know what they are doing but charge ahead as if they do. Often they are misled by fads, foolishly following their pet theories rather than learning from their patients. They overdiagnose because they see (or imagine) only the sickness in their patients and are oblivious to the health. Mistakes are also frequent when diagnoses are made casually by the undertrained and unqualified. Psychiatric diagnosis is a serious business with major and often lifelong consequences. It requires training, experience, time, empathy, and (above all) modesty.

Done well, psychiatric diagnosis can be the life-changing beginning of a successful treatment. The key ingredients to getting it right are not mysterious: a clinician with appropriate training, experience, and people skills; a patient who presents an honest and thorough description of problems; the development of a positive therapeutic relationship between them; and sufficient time to explore the past and see how things are developing in the present. If the situation is unclear, definitive diagnosis should be postponed—uncertainty is far better than false certainty. A diagnosis should always be careful—arrived at after thorough consideration, backed by solid evidence, and amenable to change as new evidence accumulates. The people helped by treatment were all confused and floundering before the moment of accurate diagnosis. Each felt helpless, unable to make sense of what was happening, uniquely damned, alone in the present, and hopeless about the future. The act of diagnosis provided a helper, an explanation, a community of fellow sufferers, a call to action, a sense of predictability, and hope for the future. Previously unmanageable problems suddenly seem manageable. An accurate diagnosis (along with education about it that is sensitive and sensible) provides great relief and a big head start toward recovery. One of the best predictors of the success of any treatment is the quality of the relationship that forms between clinician and patient. A great relationship certainly doesn't guarantee a quick cure and a lousy one doesn't foreclose it, but on average the better the relationship, the better the result. And a well-done diagnosis is one of the best ways of cementing a solid therapeutic relationship.

EPILOGUE

God must have an inordinate love of beetles because he
created so many different kinds of them.
J. B. S. HALDANE

BEETLES WILL ALMOST certainly inherit the earth. Think of the scorecard—several hundred thousand, highly diversified species of beetle versus only one increasing homogenized type of man. The smart money has to be on the bugs—not their betters—to survive to the end of our young millennium.

Nature has rolled these dice trillions and trillions of times and has learned to pick diversity as the best long-term bet. An acre of rain forest has hundreds of different species with wildly different genetic heritages. All the trees look alike to the untrained eye as they struggle to gain their little place in the sun at the top of the canopy. It would have been far less complicated to go with one species, but nature has consistently been willing to pay a hefty price to keep its options open. You never know what's coming down the pike and which genetic potential will be most needed to meet the next environmental challenge.

Nature takes the long view, mankind the short. Nature picks diversity; we pick standardization. We are homogenizing our crops and homogenizing our people. Ignoring the cautionary tale of the rain forest, mankind is now staking its destiny on a really bad bet promoted by Big Agriculture. Our food supply, once so heterogeneous, now depends on a vast global monoculture of genetically homogeneous plants and animals. Learning nothing whatever from the nightmares of the Irish potato famine, we are discounting nature's abundant and proven powers to come up with an aggressive bug that will eat our collective lunch.

And Big Pharma seems intent on pursuing a parallel attempt to create its own brand of human monoculture. With an assist from an overly ambitious psychiatry, all human difference is being transmuted into chemical imbalance that is meant to be treated with a handy pill. Turning difference into illness was among the great strokes of marketing genius accomplished in our time—up there with Apple and Facebook. But much less helpful, much more potentially harmful.

I once saw a piece of conceptual art that bore a really chilling *Brave New World* message. The artist had painstakingly measured all the wavelengths reflected off a richly detailed and brilliantly chromatic Renaissance painting. Averaging these wavelengths, she used the color that represented their mean to paint a large monochromatic canvas in what could only be described as excremental brown. It is that easy to wash out vivid difference, but how dreary the result. All the great characters in myths, novels, and plays have endured the test of time precisely because they drift so colorfully away from the mean. Do we really want to put Oedipus on the couch, give Hamlet a quick course of behavior therapy, start Lear on antipsychotics?

I think not. Human diversity has its purposes or it would not have survived the evolutionary rat race. Our ancestors made it because the tribe combined a wide variety of talents and inclinations. There were leaders high on their own narcissism and followers content enough to be dependent on them; people who were paranoid enough to sniff out hidden threats, compulsive enough to get the job done, and exhibitionistic enough to attract mates. It was good to have some who would avoid dangers, others who could ruthlessly exploit them. Perhaps the healthiest individuals were those who best balanced all these traits somewhere near the golden mean, but the best bet for the group was to have outliers always ready to step up to the plate as the particular occasion demanded. Just like all those different species of beetles and trees in the rain forest.

Darwin quickly tumbled to the idea that our brain functioning, and the human behaviors it produces, is just as much the product of natural selection as are the shape of our bodies and the workings of our digestive system. To understand ourselves, he suggested we study baboons, not books of philosophy or psychology. And he watched his children develop day to day with the practiced eye of a brilliantly thorough naturalist. He understood that if we are capable of sadness, anxiety, panic, disgust, or rage—it is because these all have high survival value and are an inevitable and existential part of human life. We need to grieve the loss of loved ones or we would never fully love them. We need to worry about the consequences of our actions or those actions will get us into trouble. We need to order our environments or chaos will ensue. Illness lurks only at the far extremes, distant from the golden mean. Most of what we do, we do for good reason. Most of us are normal.

I like eccentricity and eccentrics. The word *eccentric* comes from Greek geometry meaning "out of center." It entered English as an astronomical description of the rotational paths of the heavenly bodies. Now it is used to describe people who are different—mostly with pejorative connotations, not often enough with admiration for their particular genius. Nature abhors homogeneity and simply adores eccentric diversity. We should celebrate the fact that most humans are at least somewhat eccentric and accept ourselves as we are, warts and all. Human difference was never meant to be reducible to an exhaustive list of diagnoses drawn carelessly from a psychiatric manual. It takes all types to make a successful tribe and a full palette of emotions to make a fully lived life. We shouldn't medicalize difference and attempt to treat it away by taking the modern-day equivalent of Huxley's soma pills. The cruelest paradox of psychiatric treatment is that those who need it most often don't get it, while those who do get it often don't need it.

So how do we save normal, preserve diversity, and achieve a more rational allocation of scarce resources? Far from an easy task, but certainly not impossible. Our professionals should act professionally and within their proper competence. Psychiatrists should stick to what they do best—treating people who have real psychiatric problems— and not expand the field to include the normal worried well, who will do just fine on their own. Primary care doctors should stick to what they do best and stop being amateur psychiatrists. Drug companies should stop acting like drug cartels, irresponsibly pushing product where it will do more harm than good. Consumer advocacy groups should advocate for their consumers, not for the group. The media should expose excessive medical claims, rather than mindlessly trumpeting them.

Do we have a realistic chance to reverse diagnostic inflation, or is the die already cast in favor of a never-ending parade of false epidemics? My rational self tells me that diagnostic inflation will win and that saving normal will lose. We opponents to inflation are too few, weak, unfunded, disorganized, and face odds that are impossibly imposing. But then I am reminded of the discouraged army in *Henry V*—"we few, we happy few, we band of brothers"—who were outmanned six to one but took heart and decisively won the battle of Agincourt. Never give up on an underdog, no matter how long the odds. Every once in a while, scrawny David does pull off the seemingly impossible, and invincible Goliath does bite the dust.

And we have a big advantage on our side—our cause is right, and right sometimes does make might. It remains reasonable to hold out some hope that common sense will eventually prevail. Who would have thought that Big Tobacco, once so seemingly invincible, could be taken down so quickly? When was the last time you were with someone dangling a cigarette? Big Pharma is clearly riding for the same kind of fall—this emperor really does have no clothes.

People and policy makers may eventually wake up to the fact that we are not a bunch of sick individuals, each of us having a bunch of psychiatric diagnoses, cumulatively constituting a sick society. This is a myth generated by an overly ambitious psychiatry and a remarkably greedy pharmaceutical industry. Most of us are normal enough and would like to stay that way.

My two goals—"saving normal" and "saving psychiatry"—are really one and the same. We can "save normal" only by "saving psychiatry," and we can save psychiatry only by containing it within its proper boundaries. The legacy of Hippocrates rings as true today as it did 2,500 years ago—be modest, know your limitations, and first do no harm.

Normal is very much worth saving. And so is psychiatry.

AFTERWORD

THE ENTHUSIASTIC RECEPTION for the hardcover version of *Saving Normal* has far exceeded my modest expectations. It received favorable reviews, was translated into twelve languages; earned two book awards, and was given extensive media coverage. Readers found the book accessible, informative, thought-provoking, controversial, and troubling—but also fun. Clearly, *Saving Normal*'s messages have struck a responsive chord—we should not be turning the ordinary problems of everyday life into mental disorders; we should not let Big Pharma seduce us into becoming a pill-popping society; and we should not be over treating people who don't really need help, while shamefully neglecting those who do.

DSM-5 (published one year ago, at about the same time as *Saving Normal*) provoked a contrasting, profoundly negative reaction. Telling criticisms came from professionals, patients, the public, and the press—just about everyone could quickly see that this emperor had no clothes. Initially I felt relieved, sensing that a discredited *DSM-5* would have fewer followers and could cause less damage. But the critiques soon went way too far—the specific panning of *DSM-5* quickly morphed into a wildly generalized broadside against the entire enterprise of psychiatry. Every possible reasonable objection (and many completely unreasonable) has been raised, greatly exaggerating psychiatry's flaws while underestimating its considerable value. You know you are in the midst of a silly season when within one week the director of the National Institute of Mental Health blasts *DSM-5* for not being biological enough, while the American and the British psychological associations both suggest that *DSM-5* be scrapped altogether for being too biological. Scientologists and other radical opponents of psychiatry have feasted on the *DSM-5* debacle, using it as centerpiece in a misleading campaign to convince people to lose all faith in psychiatry. The most extreme claims are that psychiatric disorders are a myth; that psychiatric treatment is ineffective and dangerous; and that psychiatrists are at worst malign and at best hapless charlatans.

The publication of *DSM-5* also stimulated a small industry of books, blogs, papers, and videos describing the joys, perils, pitfalls, and history of psychiatric diagnosis. By far the most detailed, entertaining, and (in its way) informative of these is *The Book of Woe* by Gary Greenberg—a rollicking, sarcastic, no-holds-barred, blow-by-blow description of the making and selling of *DSM-5*. Greenberg is an energetic and perceptive participant/observer who spent several years totally immersed in the nuts and bolts of everything related to *DSM-5*. He managed to interview the major players and critics and read the relevant documents past and present. I like Gary a lot, but I don't like his book. He gets the facts of the story right but draws a one-sidedly cynical conclusion—that *DSM-5* being a mess proves that all of psychiatry is equally a mess.

I have been tireless in exposing the weak spots and harms of psychiatry. After a long career observing the errors made by others and also making my own share of mistakes, I know the weaknesses and limitations of the field perhaps as well as anyone. But I also know how helpful psychiatry can be. During my forty-year career, I have seen many dozens of patients badly harmed by psychiatric care and many hundreds not helped by it one bit. But I have also seen many thousands for whom accurate diagnosis and effective treatment have been essential to a good life, sometimes a life saver. And I have witnessed the shameful tragedy of one million psychiatric patients imprisoned for minor nuisance crimes committed because they had no access to treatment in the community and no decent place to sleep at night. We mustn't ignore the warnings of those who are critical of and/or feel harmed by psychiatry. They goad us appropriately to higher standards of practice and to greater caution, humility, and specificity of care. But the crisis of confidence caused by *DSM-5* should not detract from the value of psychiatry nor blind us to its necessity.

The only positive consequence of the *DSM-5* mess has been the heated discussions and sincere soul-searching it has stimulated (in journals, at conferences, in the media, and on the internet). Professionals and the public are engaged in an active and mostly fruitful exchange on the crucial questions of what is a mental disorder (and what is not) and when medication is necessary (and when it is harmful). Sometimes it takes going down some really dumb blind alleys before you find the right path forward. I hope that *DSM-5* represents a bottom for psychiatry and that we will now experience an upward correction. I also hope that readers of *Saving Normal* will come away with a balanced view—highly critical of psychiatry when it is done poorly, respectful of it when it is done well.

DSM-5 couldn't have caused such a big fuss if psychiatric diagnosis hadn't become so (perhaps too) important, both to individuals and to our society. It will influence all sorts of decisions—like who gets treatment and who pays for it; who qualifies for life insurance, adopting a child, flying a plane, or owning a gun; who is eligible for disability and extra school services; who gets what damages in a civil suit; whether someone goes to jail or a hospital after committing a crime; how large drug company profits and health care costs will be; and it goes on and on. Unfortunately, there is no obvious bright line helping us demarcate the inherently fuzzy boundary separating the well from the ill. Decisions are always at least somewhat arbitrary—seemingly small changes can have powerful, unpredictable, and harmful unintended consequences.

Drug companies wait on the sidelines, eager to exploit all the possible openings DSM-5 may provide. DSM-5 has fallen into the trap, making many reckless decisions that will encourage a drug-company feeding frenzy. Selling psychiatric disorders is key to selling psychiatric drugs and psychiatric drugs have become one of Big Pharma's biggest cash cows—totaling more than fifty billion dollars a year in US sales alone. The sad truth is that drug companies are lots better at selling diseases than at creating better drugs for treating them. Numerous critics charge that the people working on DSM-5 loosened the definitions of mental disorders in order to generate new customers for Pharma. I don't believe this at all. The DSM-5 experts meant well and were trying to help patients, not drug companies. But they were naive about the skill and ruthlessness of drug companies and greatly underestimated their power to mislead patients and doctors. I greatly mistrust the judgment of people working on DSM-5— but not their integrity.

Case in point: DSM-5 has made it much easier to give and to get the diagnosis of Attention Deficit Hyperactivity Disorder. The experts making this decision loosened the definition because they worried about missed cases, especially in adults. But they failed to consider that rates of Attention Deficit Disorder have already soared—so that now an astounding 20% of teenage boys get the diagnosis and 10% are on medication for it. In 1990, there were 600,000 kids on ADHD meds; now there are 3,500,000. Stimulant drugs that twenty years ago had annual revenues in the tens of millions are now approaching sales of ten billion a year. Positive proof that ADHD is way overdone comes from studies showing that the best predictor for having the diagnosis is your birthday—the youngest kid in the class is almost twice as likely to be tagged with ADHD as the eldest. Does it really make sense to turn immaturity into a mental disorder? Wouldn't it be better for our kids and our society if we spent most of those big bucks on smaller class sizes and more gym periods?

And it gets worse. A lively illegal market of diverted ADHD drugs (originally prescribed by doctors) supplies 30% of college students and 10% of high school kids with uppers for recreation and performance enhancement. Under the new, loose *DSM-5* definition of ADHD, any adult who wants to can easily get a physician to make the diagnosis and prescribe the pills. This generous market expansion will be great for Pharma shareholders and executives but bad for the many people who will be harmed by careless diagnosing and inappropriate medication. If, as a society, we want to legalize stimulants, let's do it openly— but let's not allow stimulants to become ubiquitously available based on fake medical diagnosis.

And it gets even worse. *DSM-5* provided yet another unintended gift to the ADHD drug makers in the form of its newly minted diagnosis, Binge Eating Disorder. Its definition requires only that the person have one binge eating episode a week for twelve weeks (I have easily topped that loose requirement almost every week for the past fifty years). It happens that ADHD drugs also frequently suppress appetite and are used by dieters for that purpose—although usually with poor results and with substantial risks. Recently, when a drug company announced that its ADHD medicine might also help to suppress binges, its stock quickly jumped on the expectation that this might gain it a new indication. The last thing the world needs now are more stimulant drugs being prescribed for fake indications—all encouraged by *DSM-5* diagnostic exuberance.

DSM-5 has gone overboard in many other directions. It has turned normal grief into Major Depressive Disorder—a nice gift to the aggressive antidepressant sales force. The expectable forgetfulness of old age will be mislabeled Minor Neurocognitive Disorder—leading to unnecessary worry, useless testing, and ineffective treatment. Temper tantrums become Disruptive Mood Dysregulation Disorder—risking that kids will inappropriately receive harmful medication. And worrying about physical symptoms becomes Somatic Symptom Disorder—tell that to the cancer or chronic pain patient.

The pressure to expand the boundary of mental illness is relentlessly pathologizing the predictable aches and pains of everyday life. During the past month alone, I have done interviews trying to contain misplaced enthusiasms for internet addiction, sex addiction, binge eating disorder, burnout, attention deficit disorder, autism, and, most ridiculous of all, Afluenza (the crazy idea that a teenager should get a light sentence for a DUI because he had grown up in an affluent household). The history of psychiatry is filled with such silly fads. Whenever everyone suddenly has a popular new disorder, probably no one does.

This leads to an important billion dollar public health question—how will Obamacare deal with the fact that *DSM-5* has increased by many millions the number of people who are diagnosed as having a mental disorder. The new health insurance law provides coverage to many people who previously had none and requires that there be parity for medical and mental disorders. Both features are highly desirable in theory, but neither guarantees a fair and clinically indicated allocation of mental health care. The bulk of resources should go to those who are really mentally ill and need them most. But the interacting combination of *DSM-5* and Obamacare could in fact have a perverse effect—diluting the definition of mental disorder (via *DSM-5*) and providing more coverage for its treatment (via Obamacare) may greatly expand the funding of the minor problems and thus exhaust the resources available for the serious problems. The mentally healthy might get even more unneeded services; the really sick could be even more deprived. When almost everyone is deemed more or less mentally ill, those who are truly ill get even more lost in the shuffle.

After outlining all its problems, *Saving Normal* cites a feasible plan for restoring a safe and sane psychiatry. Figuring out what to do is the easy part, but making it happen is almost impossible. Overcoming all the vested interests that benefit from the current mess will be a David vs. Goliath struggle. Fortunately, the fight against overdiagnosis in psychiatry has new allies from the much bigger and better organized fight against overdiagnosis in all the rest of medicine.

The evidence is compelling that we in the developed countries (especially the US) are over-testing for medical illness, overdiagnosing, and overtreating. Wasteful medical care of milder or nonexistent problems does more harm than good to the individual patient, diverts scarce medical resources away from those who really need them, and is an unsustainable drain on the economy. Psychiatry is therefore not alone in its groping efforts to save normal. With very few exceptions, the early screening and intervention touted by preventive medicine has turned out to be an oversold, dangerous, and expensive flop.

Routine PSA screening for prostate cancer is the clearest example. It used to be recommended that men of a certain age be tested yearly. It is now recommended that the test not be done at all unless a man has a family history or other special risk factors.

Why the big change? Definitive long-term studies prove that the test doesn't save lives and instead ruins them by triggering invasive interventions with painful complications. Screening is usually too late to stop fast spreading tumors and too good at identifying slow-growing ones that don't count and are better left alone. If they live long enough, the majority of men will develop an incidental and benign prostate cancer before they die from something else. Picking up these tumors early causes a great deal of grief for no return.

Lowering the thresholds of disease definitions has identified diseases that don't exist—fake hypertension, fake diabetes, fake osteoporosis, and so on. The hopeful dream was that getting there early would help prevent the development of severe heart problems, hypertension, diabetes, osteoporosis, and a score of other illnesses. The painful reality is that getting there too early misidentifies too many people who are not really at risk and then subjects them to needless and harmful tests and treatments.

Medical technology has gotten out of hand. If we do enough CT scans we can find structural abnormalities in just about everyone. But most findings are incidental and don't have any real clinical meaning. Paradoxically, lots of otherwise healthy people will get dangerous cancers from the CT radiation that served no useful purpose.

Doctors have gotten into the habit of ordering huge batteries of tests and treating the lab results while ignoring what is best for this particular patient. There needs to be retraining of those already in practice, a change in how medicine is taught to new doctors, and a realignment of financial incentives to promote best care, not excessive care. As in psychiatry, we should protect the really well from getting what is often excessive and harmful care and should provide more resources to treat the really sick. It is wonderful that medical knowledge and tools have advanced so far, but disheartening that we are so bad at distributing them rationally.

Curing excess in all of medicine will not be easy. Harmful over-testing and overtreating is promoted and protected by the enormous economic and political power of the medical industrial complex. A great deal of progress has already been made. Fifty medical professional associations in the US have seen the need to cut back on inappropriate testing and treatment. Their "Choosing Wisely" initiative is a terrific start in reforming the disaster of our medical nonsystem. *The British Medical Journal* and *Consumers' Reports* have played a catalytic role and are powerful platforms for spreading the evidence to physicians and patients. People need to become smarter consumers and not buy into the idea that more is always better.

In this David vs. Goliath struggle, the forces that benefit from massive overdiagnosis can marshal hundreds of billions of dollars a year to promote and protect it. The forces supporting rational medical decision making have access to just a few million dollars a year. The smart money is betting on the big bucks and the status quo. But there is hope. Big Tobacco also seemed impregnable just twenty-five years ago but was brought down by hard facts and a tiny band of dedicated reformers. Right sometimes does bring might. And I hope that *Saving Normal* does its small part in furthering common sense in psychiatry and medicine.

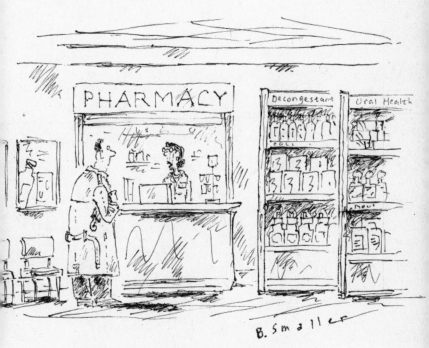

"That would be in Aisle Six, the worried-well section."

ACKNOWLEDGMENTS

Aʟᴍᴏsᴛ ᴀʟʟ ᴏғ what I know about psychiatry (and also much of what I know about life, people, and myself) has come from my patients. Thanks to them and also to the eighteen people who contributed moving memoirs describing their sometimes dreadful, sometimes wonderful experiences with psychiatric diagnosis and treatment. Then there are the hundreds of colleagues who have helped me in so many ways during my career in psychiatry. I can't possibly thank you all by name, but you know who you are and that I am forever and deeply grateful. There are just a few specific people I must mention. Being by nature a selfish and fun-loving person, I would not have taken on willingly the difficult burden of reforming psychiatry—especially at this late and otherwise duty-free point in my life. My hand was forced by the shaming example of several of my betters. Bob Spitzer got me started in the diagnostic game thirty-five years ago and has spent most of his waking life devoted to improving it. Barney Carroll's tireless efforts to hold psychiatry to the highest standards forced me to step up to the plate when I saw our field falling short of them. He doesn't know it, but Paul McHugh's many courageous stands also influenced me not to just sit tight enjoying the beach. And although I strongly disagreed with the extremist views of the recently deceased Tom Szasz, I very much liked him personally and always admired his willingness to fight for what he thought was right, regardless of personal sacrifice. The example of my greathearted friend Yutaka Ono helped me to make the book more personal and less stilted than comes naturally to me. Suzy Chapman has done us all and history a great service by archiving a vast trove of *DSM-5* and *ICD-11* documents. Gary Greenberg has written a wonderful "Book of Woe" describing the *DSM-5* follies. I also give special thanks to my ragtag pickup team of Internet buddies (many of whom I have never met) who helped me sort out the *DSM-5* mess and contributed ideas to this book—especially Melissa Raven, Mickey Nardo, Dayle Jones, Joanne Cacciatore, Donna Rockwell, Russell Friedman, Marianne Russo, Martin Whitely, Jon Jureidini, Chris Kane, Margaret Soltana, and James Phillips. My usually noisy grandchildren displayed surprising and uncharacteristic forbearance as I spent seemingly endless hours typing out and editing this book on my beloved BlackBerry—which they delight in calling "my evil friend." My agent, Carrie Kania, not only sold the book—she also helped conceive it and gave it shape. My American editor, Peter Hubbard; my German editor, Laurenz Bolliger; and my Dutch editor, Michiel ten Raa, all made numerous and important suggestions. And most important of all, my wife, Donna—a great reader who made me a better writer.

NOTES

PREFACE

1. Medco, "America's State of Mind" (2011). http://www.toxicpsychiatry.com/storage/Psych%20Drug%20Us%20Epidemic%20Medco%20rpt%Nov%20 2011.pdf.
2. S. H. Zuvekas and B. Vitiello, "Stimulant Medication Use in Children: A 12-Year Perspective," *Am J Psychiatry* 169, no. 2 (2012).
3. B. Vitiello, S. H. Zuvekas, and G. S. Norquist, "National Estimates of Antidepressant Medication Use Among U.S. Children, 1997–2002," *J Am Acad Child Adolesc Psychiatry* 45, no. 3 (2006).
4. G. Epstein-Lubow and A. Rosenzweig, "The Use of Antipsychotic Medication in Long-Term Care," *Med Health R I* 93, no. 12 (2010).
5. T. Pringsheim, D. Lam, and S. B. Patten, "The Pharmacoepidemiology of Antipsychotic Medications for Canadian Children and Adolescents: 2005–2009," *J Child Adolesc Psychopharmacol* 21, no. 6 (2011).
6. Centers for Disease Control and Prevention, "Prescription Painkiller Overdoses at Epidemic Levels,"(2011); http://www.cdc.gov/media/releases/2011/p1101_flu_pain_killer_overdose.html.
7. Kim Murphy, "A Fog of Drugs and War," *Los Angeles Times,* April 7, 2012, accessed September 16, 2012; http://articles.latimes.com/2012/apr/07/nation/la-na-army-medication-20120408.
8. IMS Institute for Health Informatics, "The Use of Medicines in the United States: Review of 2011" (2012).
9. M.N. Stagnitti, "Trends in the Use and Expenditures for the Therapeutic Class Prescribed Psychotherapeutic Agents and All Subclasses, 1997 and 2004" (2007).
10. Laura A. Pratt, Debra J. Brody, and Qiuping Gu, "Antidepressant Use in Persons Aged 12 and Over: United States, 2005–2008," in NCHS Data Brief (Hyattsville, MD, 2011).
11. T. L. Mark, K. R. Levit, and J. A. Buck, "Datapoints: Psychotropic Drug Prescriptions by Medical Specialty," *Psychiatr Serv* 60, no. 9 (2009).
12. Stefan Leucht, "Putting the efficacy of psychiatric and general medicine medication into perspective: review of meta-analyses," *British Journal of Psychiatry* 200, (2012): 97–106 doi: 10.1192/bjp.bp.111.096594.

CHAPTER ONE

1. *Oxford English Dictionary,* Oxford University Press, http://oxforddictionaries.com/definition/english/normal (2012).
2. Jeremy Bentham, *Utilitarianism* (London: Progressive Publishing Company, 1890).

3. Jagdish K. Patel and Campbell B. Read, *Handbook of the Normal Distribution* (New York: Marcel Dekker, Inc., 1996).

4. Vivian Nutton, *Ancient Medicine* (New York: Routledge, 2004).

5. Preamble to the Constitution of the World Health Organization as adopted by the International Health Conference, New York, June 19–22, 1946; signed on 22 July 1946 by the representatives of 61 States (Official Records of the World Health Organization, no. 2, p. 100) and entered into force on 7 April 1948. The definition has not been amended since 1948.

6. ABIM Foundation, "Choosing Wisely"; http://www.abimfoundation.org/Initiatives/Choosing-Wisely.aspx (accessed August 18, 2012).

7. "Neuron,"http://en.wikipedia.org/wiki/Neuron#Neurons_in_the_brain (accessed August 18, 2012).

8. "Roger W. Sperry—Nobel Lecture: Some Effects of Disconnecting the Cerebral Hemispheres." Nobelprize.org. 26 Sep 2012; http://www.nobelprize.org/nobel_prizes/medicine/laureates/1981/sperry-lecture.htm.

9. N. J. Macintosh, *I.Q. and Human Intelligence* (New York: Oxford University Press, 1998).

10. *Atkins v. Virginia* (00-8452) 536 U.S. 304 (2002) 260 Va. 375, 534 S.E. 2D 312.

11. Emile Durkheim, George Simpson, and John A. Spaulding, *Suicide* (New York: The Free Press, 1951).

12. Sigmund Freud, *An Outline of Psychoanalysis* (New York: W. W. Norton 1949).

13. Jerome Wakefield, "The concept of mental disorder: On the boundary between biological facts and social values," *American Psychologist,* 47 (1992): 373–88.

14. R. M. Bergner, "What is psychopathology? And so what?" *Clin Psychol Sci Pract.* 4 (1997): 235–48.

15. D. F. Klein, "Harmful dysfunction, disorder, disease, illness, and evolution," *J Abnorm Psychol* 108 (1999): 421–29.

16. T. A. Widiger and L. M. Sankis, "Adult psychopathology: issues and controversies," *Annu Rev Psychol* 51 (2000): 377–404

17. J. C. Wakefield and M. B. First, "Clarifying the distinction between disorder and nondisorder: confronting the overdiagnosis (false-positives) problem in *DSM-V*," In *Advancing DSM. Dilemmas in Psychiatric Diagnosis,* ed. K. A. Phillips, M. B. First, H. A. Pincus (Washington, D.C.: American Psychiatric Association, 2003), 23–55.

18. *Diagnostic and Statistical Manual of Mental Disorders* (4th ed., text rev.) (Washington, D.C.: American Psychiatric Press, 2000).

19. R. L. Spitzer and J. B. W. Williams, "The definition and diagnosis of mental disorder," In *Deviance and Mental Illness,* ed. W. R. Gove (Beverly Hills, CA: Sage, 1982), 15–32.

20. D. J. Stein and others, "What is a mental/psychiatric disorder? From *DSM-IV* to *DSM-V*." *Psychol Med* 40 (2010): 1759–65.

21. J. C. Wakefield, "The myth of *DSM*'s invention of new categories of disorder: Hout's diagnostic discontinuity thesis disconfirmed," *Behav Res Ther* 39 (2001): 575–624.

22. S. A. Kirk, ed., *Mental Disorders in the Social Environment: Critical Perspectives* (New York: Columbia University Press, 2005).

23. Jeffrey A. Schaler and others, "Mental Health and the Law," *Cato Unbound*, August 12, 2012 edition; http://www.cato-unbound.org/issues/august-2012-mental-health-and-the-law.

24. James Phillips and others, "The Six Most Essential Questions in Psychiatric Diagnosis," *Philosophy, Ethics and Humanities in Medicine*, February 2012; http://www.peh-med.com/content/7/1/3.

25. D. S. Charney and others, "Neuroscience research agenda to guide development of a pathophysiologically based classification system," in *A Research Agenda for DSM-V*, eds. D. J. Kupfer, M. B. First, D. A. Regier (Washington, D.C.: American Psychiatric Association, 2005), 31–84.

26. S. Hyman, "The diagnosis of mental disorders: the problem of reification," *Annu Rev Clin Psychol.* 6 (2010):155–79.

27. T. R. Insel, "Translating scientific opportunity into public health impact. A strategic plan for research on mental illness," *Arch Gen Psychiatry* 66 (2009): 128–33.

28. K. S. Kendler, "Toward a philosophical structure for psychiatry," *Am J Psychiatry* 162 (2005): 433–40.

29. J. Paris, "Endophenotypes and the diagnosis of personality disorders," *J Personal Disord* 25 (2011): 260–68.

30. T. Szasz, *The Myth of Mental Illness: Foundations of a Theory of Personal Conduct* (New York: Harper & Row, 1974).

31. M. B. First and A. J. Frances, "Issues for *DSM-V*: unintended consequences of small changes: the case of paraphilias," *Am J Psychiatry* 165 (2008): 1240–41.

32. A. J. Frances and others, "*DSM-IV*: work in progress," *Am J Psychiatry* 147 (1990): 1439–48.

33. A. Barnes, "Race, schizophrenia, and admission to state psychiatric hospitals," *Administration and Policy in Mental Health* 31 (2004): 241–52.

34. *ICD-10 Classifications of Mental and Behavioural Disorder: Clinical Descriptions and Diagnostic Guidelines* (Geneva: World Health Organisation, 1992).

35. A. Frances, "Integrating *DSM-5* and ICD 11," *Psychiatric Times*, November 2009.

36. Richard Dawkins, *The Ancestor's Tale: A Pilgrimage to the Dawn of Evolution* (Boston: Houghton Mifflin, 2004), 416.

37. Paul R. McHugh, MD, and Phillip R. Slavney, MD, "Comprehensive Evaluation or Checklist?" *New England J Med* 366, no. 20 (2012): 1853–55.

CHAPTER TWO

1. Genesis 2:20, Holy Bible, King James Version (Cambridge Edition, 2000).

2. *Encyclopaedia Britannica*, online edition, 2012, s.v. "Shamanism," http://www.britannica.com/EBchecked/topic/538200/shamanism.

3. Jerome D. Frank and Julia B. Frank, *Persuasion and Healing: A Comparative Study of Psychotherapy* (Baltimore: The Johns Hopkins University Press, 1961).

4. M. Fornaro, N. Clementi, and P. Fornaro, "Medicine and Psychiatry in Western Culture: Ancient Greek Myths and Modern Prejudices," *Ann Gen Psychiatry* 8 (2009): 21.

5. Hippocrates, *The Corpus: The Hippocratic Writings* (New York: Kaplan, 2008).

6. Galen (edited and translated by Ian Johnson), *On Symptoms and Disease* (Cambridge, U.K.: Cambridge University Press, 2011).

7. Roy Porter, *Madness: A Brief History* (Oxford, U.K.: Oxford University Press, 2002).

8. Heinrich Kramer and James Sprenger (translated by Christopher Mackay), *Malleus Maleficarum* (Cambridge, U.K.: Cambridge University Press, 2006).

9. "Medicine in the Medieval Islamic World," Wikipedia, last modified August 18, 2012, http://en.wikipedia.org/wiki/Medicine_in_the_medieval_Islamic_world.

10. Joseph Frank Payne, *Thomas Sydenham* (Charleston, SC: Nabu Press, 2010).

11. Wilfrid Blunt, *Linnaeus, the Complete Naturalist* (Princeton, NJ: Princeton University Press, 2001).

12. Jan E. Goldstein, *Console and Classify: The French Psychiatric Profession in the Nineteenth Century* (Chicago: University of Chicago Press, 1987).

13. E. Shorter, *A History of Psychiatry: From the Era of the Asylum to the Age of Prozac* (New York: John Wiley, 1997).

14. Hans Pols, PhD, and Stephanie Oak, BMed, "War and Military Mental Health," *Am J Public Health* 97, no. 12 (2007): 2132–42.

15. Walter E. Barton, MD, *History and Influence of the American Psychiatric Association* (Washington, D.C.: American Psychiatric Association Press, 1987).

16. *DSM-I: Diagnostic and Statistical Manual of Mental Disorders* (American Psychiatric Association, 1952).

17. *DSM-II: Diagnostic and Statistical Manual of Mental Disorders* (Washington D.C., American Psychiatric Association, 1968).

18. John E. Cooper and others, "Cross-National Study of the Mental Disorders: Some Results from the First Comparative Investigation," *Am J Psychiatry* 125 (1969): 21–29.

19. R. L. Spitzer, J. Endicott, and E. Robins, *Research Diagnostic Criteria (RDC) for a Selected Group of Functional Disorders*, 3rd ed. (New York State Psychiatric Institute, 1978).

20. J. Endicott and R. L. Spitzer, "A diagnostic interview: the schedule for affective disorders and schizophrenia," *Arch Gen Psychiatry* 35 (1978): 35, 773–82.

21. *DSM-III: Diagnostic and Statistical Manual of Mental Disorders*, 3rd ed. (Washington, D.C.: American Psychiatric Association, 1985).

22. H. H. Decker, *The Making of DSM-III: A Diagnostic Manual's Conquest of American Psychiatry* (Oxford, U.K.: Oxford University Press, 2013).

23. *DSM-IIIR: Diagnostic and Statistical Manual of Mental Disorders*, 3rd ed., rev. (Washington, D.C.: American Psychiatric Association, 1987).

24. *DSM-IV: Diagnostic and Statistical Manual of Mental Disorders* (Washington, D.C.: American Psychiatric Association, 1994).

25. A. J. Frances, T. A. Widiger, and H. A. Pincus, "The development of *DSM-IV*," *Arch Gen Psychiatry* 6 (1989): 373–75.

26. Thomas A. Widiger, PhD, and Allen J. Frances, MD, *DSM-IV* Sourcebook, volumes 1–4 (Washington, D.C.: American Psychiatric Press, 1994).

27. A. J. Frances, M. B. First, and H. A. Pincus, *DSM-IV* Guidebook (Washington, D.C.: American Psychiatric Press, 1995).

28. A. J. Frances and others, "*DSM-IV*: work in progress," *Am J Psychiatry* 147 (1990): 1439–48.

29. L. Cosgrove, S. Krimsky (2012) "A Comparison of *DSM-IV* and *DSM-5* Panel Members' Financial Associations with Industry: A Pernicious Problem Persists," *PLoS Med* 9(3): e1001190. doi:10.1371/journal.pmed.1001190.

30. L. Cosgrove, H. J. Bursztajn, and S. Krimsky, "Developing unbiased diagnostic and treatment guidelines in psychiatry," *N Eng J Med* 360 (2009): 2035–36.

CHAPTER THREE

1. R. Moynihan, J. Doust, and D. Henry, "Preventing Overdiagnosis: How to Stop Harming the Healthy," *BMJ* 344 (2012): e3502.

2. "Choosing Wisely: Five Things Physicians and Patients Should Question" (2012) ABIM Foundation, http://choosingwisely.org/?page_id=13.

3. Paul Enright, "A Homeopathic Remedy for Early COPD," *Respiratory Medicine* 105 (2011): 1573–75.

4. U.S. Preventive Services Task Force, "Screening for Breast Cancer: U.S. Preventive Services Task Force Recommendation Statement," *Ann Intern Med* 151, no. 10 (2009): 716–26.

5. R. Harris, "Overview of Screening: Where We Are and Where We May Be Headed," *Epidemiologic Reviews* 33, no. 1 (2011): 1–6.

6. Andrew J Bacevich, "The Tyranny of Defense Inc.," *The Atlantic* (January/February 2011) http://www.theatlantic.com/magazine/archive/2011/01/the-tyranny-of-defense-inc/308342.

7. Organisation for Economic Co-operation and Development, "Why Is Health Spending in the United States So High?"(2011); http://www.oecd.org/unitedstates/49084355.pdf.

8. P. D. McGorry, "Is Early Intervention in the Major Psychiatric Disorders Justified? Yes," *BMJ* 337 (2008): a695.

9. Brian Deer, "How the Case Against the MMR Vaccine Was Fixed," *BMJ* 342 (2011), http://www.bmj.com/content/342/bmj.c5347.

10. L. Batstra and others, "Childhood Emotional and Behavioral Problems: Reducing Overdiagnosis Without Risking Undertreatment," *Dev Med Child Neurol* 54, no. 6 (2012): 492–94.

11. R. L. Morrow and others, "Influence of Relative Age on Diagnosis and Treatment of Attention-Deficit/Hyperactivity Disorder in Children," *CMAJ* 184, no. 7 (2012): 755–62.

12. Peter Parry, "Paediatric Bipolar Disorder (Pbd) and Pre-Pubertal Paediatric Bipolar Disorder (PPBD)—a Controversy from America," (2009) Black Dog Institute,http://www.blackdoginstitute.org.au/docs/PaediatricbipolardisoderacontroversyfromtheUSA.pdf.

13. A. Frances, Editorial: "Problems in Defining Clinical Significance in Epidemiological Studies," *Arch Gen Psychiatry* 55, no. 2 (1998): 119.

14. Substance Abuse and Mental Health Services Administration, "Results from the 2009 National Survey on Drug Use and Health: Mental Health Findings," (Rockville, MD, 2012).

15. Peter D. Kramer, *Listening to Prozac* (New York: Penguin, 1993).

16. S. J. Williams, P. Martin, and J. Gabe, "The Pharmaceuticalisation of Society? A Framework for Analysis," *Sociol Health Illn* 33, no. 5 (2011): 710–25.

17. Rick Newman, "Why Health Insurers Make Lousy Villains," *US News & World Report*, Money Section, August 25, 2009, accessed September 25, 2012;

http://money.usnews.com/money/blogs/flowchart/2009/08/25/why-health-insurers-make-lousy-villains.

18. M. A. Gagnon and J. Lexchin, "The Cost of Pushing Pills: A New Estimate of Pharmaceutical Promotion Expenditures in the United States," *PLoS Med* 5, no. 1 (2008), http://www.plosmedicine.org/article/info:doi/10.1371/journal.pmed.0050001.

19. Jeffrey Lieberman and others, "Effects of Antipsychotic Drugs in Patients with Schizophrenia," *New England J Med* 353 (September 22, 2005): 1209–33.

20. F. S. Sierles and others, "Medical Students' Exposure to and Attitudes About Drug Company Interactions: A National Survey," *JAMA* 294, no. 9 (2005): 1034–42.

21. R. Mojtabai and M. Olfson, "National Trends in Psychotropic Medication Polypharmacy in Office-Based Psychiatry," *Arch Gen Psychiatry* 67, no. 1 (2010).

22. J. S. Comer, M. Olfson, and R. Mojtabai, "National Trends in Child and Adolescent Psychotropic Polypharmacy in Office-Based Practice, 1996–2007," *J Am Acad Child Adolesc Psychiatry* 49, no. 10 (2010).

23. Substance Abuse and Mental Health Services Administration, "Results from the 2011 National Survey on Drug Use and Health: Summary of National Findings," NSDUH Series H-41, HHS Publication No. (SMA) 11-4658. Rockville, MD: Substance Abuse and Mental Health Services Administration, 2012.

24. Tracy Staton and Eric Palmer, "Pharma's Top 11 Marketing Settlements" Fierce Pharma (June 26, 2012) http://www.fiercepharma.com/special-reports/top-10-pharma-settlements/top-10-pharma-settlements.

25. Bill Berkrot and Pierson Randell, "J&J to Pay $181 Mln to Settle Improper Marketing Claims," Thomson Reuters News & Insights, August 30, 2012, http://www.reuters.com/article/2012/08/30/us-johnsonandjohnson-settlement-idUSBRE87T10X20120830.

26. Department of Justice, "GlaxoSmithKline to Plead Guilty and Pay $3 Billion to Resolve Fraud Allegations and Failure to Report Safety Data" (2012); http://www.justice.gov/opa/pr/2012/July/12-civ-842.html.

27. Department of Justice, "Abbott Labs to Pay $1.5 Billion to Resolve Criminal Civil Investigations of Off-Label Promotion of Depakote" (2012); http://www.justice.gov/opa/pr/2012/May/12-civ-585.html.

28. Bill Berkrot and Pierson Randell, "J&J to Pay $181 Mln to Settle Improper Marketing Claims," Thomson Reuters News & Insights, August 30, 2012, http://www.reuters.com/article/2012/08/30/us-johnsonandjohnson-settlement-idUSBRE87T10X20120830.

29. Ed Silverman, "After the Risperdal Trial, J&J Looks More Like Humpty-Dumpty," *Forbes*, 20 January 2012, http://www.forbes.com/sites/edsilverman/2012/01/20/after-the-risperdal-trial-jj-looks-more-like-humpty-dumpty.

30. Department of Justice, "Novartis Pharmaceuticals Corp. to Pay More Than $420 Million to Resolve Off-Label Promotion and Kickback Allegations" (2010); http://www.justice.gov/opa/pr/2010/September/10-civ-1102.html.

31. Department of Justice, "Drug Maker Forest Pleads Guilty; to Pay More Than $313 Million to Resolve Criminal Charges and False Claims Act Allegations," (2010); http://www.justice.gov/opa/pr/2010/September/10-civ-1028.html.

32. Department of Justice, "Pharmaceutical Giant AstraZeneca to Pay $520 Million for Off-Label Drug Marketing" (2010); http://www.justice.gov/opa/pr/2010/April/10-civ-487.html.

33. Department of Justice, "Pfizer to Pay $2.3 Billion for Fraudulent Marketing" (2009); http://www.justice.gov/opa/pr/2009/September/09-civ-900.html.

34. Department of Justice, "Eli Lilly and Company Agrees to Pay $1.415 Billion to Resolve Allegations of Off-Label Promotion of Zyprexa" (2009); http://www.justice.gov/opa/pr/2009/January/09-civ-038.html.

35. Department of Justice, "The Accomplishments of the U.S. Department of Justice 2001–2009" (2009), http://www.fas.org/irp/agency/doj/2001-2009.pdf.

36. Department of Justice, "Justice Department Recovers $2 Billion for Fraud Against the Government in Fy 2007; More Than $20 Billion since 1986" (2007); http://www.justice.gov/opa/pr/2007/November/07_civ_873.html.

37. Department of Justice, "Warner-Lambert to Pay $430 Million to Resolve Criminal & Civil Health Care Liability Relating to Off-Label Promotion" (2004); http://www.justice.gov/opa/pr/2004/May/04_civ_322.htm.

38. J. C. Fournier and others, "Antidepressant Drug Effects and Depression Severity: A Patient-Level Meta-Analysis," *JAMA* 303, no. 1 (2010).

39. I. Kirsch, "Antidepressants and the Placebo Response," *Epidemiological Psychiatr Soc* 18, no. 4 (2009): 318–22.

40. M. Fassler and others, "Frequency and Circumstances of Placebo Use in Clinical Practice—a Systematic Review of Empirical Studies," *BMC Med* 8 (2010); http://www.biomedcentral.com/1741-7015/8/15.

41. Laura A. Pratt, Debra J. Brody, and Qiuping Gu, "Antidepressant Use in Persons Aged 12 and Over: United States, 2005–2008," in *NCHS Data Brief* (Hyattsville, MD, 2011).

42. Ryan Du Bosar, "Psychotropic Drug Prescriptions by Medical Specialty," *ACP Internist* (2009), http://www.acpinternist.org/archives/2009/11/national-trends.htm.

43. Leslie Russell, "Mental Health Care Services in Primary Care," monograph, Center for American Progress (October, 2010); http://www.americanprogress.org/issues/healthcare/report/2010/10/04/8466/mental-health-care-services-in-primary-care.

44. Peter J. Cunningham, "Beyond Parity: Primary Care Physicians' Perspective on Access to Mental Health Care," *Health Affairs* 28, no. 3 (May/June 2009): 490–501; doi: 10.1377/hlthaff.28.3.w490.

45. L. N. Robins and others, "Lifetime Prevalence of Specific Psychiatric Disorders in Three Sites," *Arch Gen Psychiatry* 41, no. 10 (1984): 949–58.

46. R. C. Kessler and others, "Lifetime Prevalence and Age-of-Onset Distributions of *DSM-IV* Disorders in the National Comorbidity Survey Replication," *Arch Gen Psychiatry* 62, no. 6 (2005): 593–602.

47. R. de Graaf and others., "Prevalence of Mental Disorders and Trends from 1996 to 2009. Results from the Netherlands Mental Health Survey and Incidence Study-2," *Soc Psychiatry Psychiatr Epidemiol* 47, no. 2 (2012): 303–13.

48. T. E. Moffitt et al., "How Common Are Common Mental Disorders? Evidence That Lifetime Prevalence Rates Are Doubled by Prospective Versus Retrospective Ascertainment," *Psychol Med* 40, no. 6 (2010): 899–909.

49. W. Copeland and others, "Cumulative Prevalence of Psychiatric Disorders by Young Adulthood: A Prospective Cohort Analysis from the Great Smoky Mountains Study," *J Am Acad Child Adolesc Psychiatry* 50, no. 3 (2011): 252–61.

50. C. Moreno, G. Laje, C. Blanco, H. Jiang, A. B. Schmidt, and M. Olfson, "National trends in the outpatient diagnosis and treatment of bipolar disorder in youth," *Arch Psychiatry* 64 (2007):1032–39.

51. CDC estimates 1 in 88 children in United States has been identified as having an autism spectrum disorder (accessed October 8, 2012); http://www.cdc.gov/media/releases/2012/p0329_autism_disorder.html.

52. B. Bloom, R. A. Cohen, and G. Freeman, "Summary health statistics for U.S. children: National Health Interview Survey, 2010," National Center for Health Statistics. Vital Health Statistics, Series 10, no. 250 (2011); http://www.cdc.gov/nchs/data/series/sr_10/sr10_250.pdf.

53. T. A. Ketter, "Diagnostic features, prevalence, and impact of bipolar disorder," *J Clin Psychiatry* 71, no. 6 (June 2010): e14.

54. Richard A. Friedman, "A Call for Caution on Antipsychotic Drugs," *New York Times*, Health Section, September 24, 2012 (accessed September 25, 2012); http://www.nytimes.com/2012/09/25/health/a-call-for-caution-in-the-use-of-antipsychotic-drugs.html?_r=1.

55. B. L. Smith, "Inappropriate Prescribing," American Psychological Association; http://www.apa.org/monitor/2012/06/prescribing.aspx (accessed September 19, 2012).

56. Michael Kleinrock, "The Use of Medications in the US: Review of 2012," IMS Institute for Health Informatics, p. 28 (accessed September 25, 2012); http://www.imshealth.com/imshealth/Global/Content/IMS%20Institute/Documents/IHII_UseOfMed_report%20.pdf.

57. Jonathan S. Comer, Ramin Mojtabai, and Mark Olfson, "National Trends in the Antipsychotic Treatment of Outpatients with Anxiety Disorders," *Am J Psychiatry* 168 (2011): 1057–65.

58. G. Caleb Alexander and others, "Increasing Off-Label Use of Antipsychotic Medications in the US, 1995–2008," National Institutes of Health (January 6, 2011); doi: 10.10021pds.2082.

59. Centers for Disease Control and Prevention, "Drug Overdose Deaths—Florida, 2003–2009," *MMWR Morb Mortal Wkly Rep* 60, no. 26 (2011).

60. Peter W. Chiarelli, "Army Health Promotion Risk Reduction Suicide Prevention Report 2010," U.S. Department of Defense, American Forces Press Service (2010), http://www.defense.gov/News/NewsArticle.aspx?ID=60236.

61. Gardiner Harris, "Talk Doesn't Pay, So Psychiatry Turns Instead to Drug Therapy," *New York Times*, March 5, 2011.

62. J. C. West and others, "Economic Grand Rounds: Financial Disincentives for the Provision of Psychotherapy," *Psychiatr Serv* 54, no. 12 (2003): 1582–83.

63. R. Mojtabai and M. Olfson, "National Patterns in Antidepressant Treatment by Psychiatrists and General Medical Providers: Results from the National Comorbidity Survey Replication," *J Clin Psychiatry* 69, no. 7 (2008): 1064–74.

64. M. W. Otto and others, "A Comparison of the Efficacy of Clonazepam and

Cognitive-Behavioral Group Therapy for the Treatment of Social Phobia," *J Anxiety Disord* 14, no. 4 (2000): 345–58.

65. B. Roshanaei-Moghaddam and others, "Relative Effects of Cbt and Pharmacotherapy in Depression Versus Anxiety: Is Medication Somewhat Better for Depression, and Cbt Somewhat Better for Anxiety?" *Depress Anxiety* 28, no. 7 (2011): 560–67.

66. G. I. Spielmans, M. I. Berman, and A. N. Usitalo, "Psychotherapy Versus Second-Generation Antidepressants in the Treatment of Depression: A Meta-Analysis," *J Nerv Ment Dis* 199, no. 3 (2011): 142–49.

67. N. R. Silton and others, "Stigma in America: Has Anything Changed? Impact of Perceptions of Mental Illness and Dangerousness on the Desire for Social Distance: 1996 and 2006," *J Nerv Ment Dis* 199, no. 6 (2011): 361–66.

68. R. Smith, "In Search of Non-Disease," BMJ 324, no. 7342 (April 13, 2002): 883–85.

69. Charles Rosenberg, *The Trial of the Assassin Guiteau* (New York: The Notable Trials Library, 1996).

70. P. S. Wang and others, "Use of Mental Health Services for Anxiety, Mood, and Substance Disorders in 17 Countries in the WHO World Mental Health Surveys," *The Lancet* 370, no. 9590 (2007): 841–50.

CHAPTER FOUR

1. Hilary Evans and Robert E. Bartholomew, *Outbreak!, The Encyclopedia of Extraordinary Social Behavior* (San Antonio, TX: Anomalist Press, 2009).

2. I. M. Lewis, *Ecstatic Religion: A Study of Shamanism and Spiritual Possession* (New York: Routledge, 2003).

3. John Waller, *The Dancing Plague: The Strange True Story of an Extraordinary Illness* (Naperville, IL: Sourcebooks, 2009).

4. Mark Collins Jenkins, *Vampire Forensics: Uncovering the Origins of an Enduring Legend* (Washington, D.C.: National Geographic Society, 2010).

5. Johann Wolfgang von Goethe (Translated and edited by Michael Hulse), *The Sorrows of Young Werther* (London, U.K.: Penguin Books, 1989).

6. CDC, "Suicide Contagion and the Reporting of Suicide; Recommendations from a National Workshop on Reporting on Suicide" (accessed August 22, 2012): www.cdc.gov/mmwr/preview/mmwrhtml/00031539.htm.

7. Isaac G. Briggs, *Epilepsy, Hysteria and Neurasthenia: Their Causes, Symptoms, Treatment* (Charleston, SC: Bibliobazaar, 2007).

8. Josef Breuer and Sigmund Freud, *Studies in Hysteria* (New York: Basic Books, 2000).

9. Harold Merskey, *The Analysis of Hysteria,* 2nd ed. (London, U.K.: The Royal College of Psychiatry, 1995).

10. Corbett H. Thigpen, MD, and Hervey Cleckley, MD, *The Three Faces of Eve* (New York: McGraw-Hill, 1957).

11. August Piper, MD, and Harold Merskey, DM, "The Persistence of Folly: A Critical Examination of Dissociative Identity Disorder Part II: The Defence and Decline of Multiple Personality or DID," *Canadian J Psychiatry* 49, no. 10 (2004): 678–83.

12. Debbie Nathan, *Satan's Silence: Ritual Abuse and the Making of a Modern American Witch Hunt* (Lincoln, NE: Author's Choice Press, 1995).

CHAPTER FIVE

1. H. A. Pincus, "*DSM-IV* and new diagnostic categories: Holding the line on proliferation," *Am J Psychiatry* 149 (1992): 112–17.

2. Laura Batstra and Allen Frances, "Diagnostic Inflation: Causes and a Suggested Cure," *Nerv Ment Disease* 200, no. 6 (June 2012): 474–79; doi: 10.1097/NMD.0b013e318257c4a2.

3. Richard L. Morrow, and others "Influence of relative age on diagnosis and treatment of attention-deficit/hyperactivity disorder in children," *CMAJ,* March 5, 2012; http://www.cmaj.ca/content/early/2012/03/05/cmaj.111619.full.pdf+html.

4. S. Boyles, "Study confirms ADHD is more common in boys," *WebMD Health News,* September 15, 2004; http://www.webmd.com/add-adhd/news/20040915/study-confirms-adhd-is-more-common-in-boys (accessed March 10, 2011).

5. K. Bruchmüller, J. Margraf, and S. Schneider, "Is ADHD Diagnosed in Accord with Diagnostic Criteria? Overdiagnosis and Influence of Client Gender on Diagnosis," *J Consult Clin Psychology* 80, no. 1 (February 2012): 128–38; doi: 10.1037/a0026582.

6. Howard Wolinsky, "Disease Mongering and Drug Marketing," *EMBO Reports* 6, no. 7 (July 2005): 612–14, accessed September 4, 2012; http://www.ncbi.nlm.nih.gov/pmc/articles/PMC1369125.

7. C. B. Phillips, "Medicine goes to school: teachers as sickness brokers for ADHD," *PLoS Med.* 3, no. 4 (2006): 433–35.

8. "Short-Supply Prescription Drugs: Shining a Light on the Gray Market," Democratic Press Office, July 25, 2012; http://commerce.senate.gov/public/index.cfm?p=Hearings&ContentRecord_id=0c41d6c9-cce9-4f59-bb82-fb19bfd057dc&ContentType_id=14f995b9-dfa5-407a-9d35-56cc7152a7ed&Group_id=b06c39af-e033-4cba-9221-de668ca1978a.

9. Martin Whitely, *Speed Up and Sit Still: The Controversies of ADHD Diagnosis and Treatment* (Perth: UWA Publishing, 2010).

10. Carmen Moreno, MD, and others, "National Trends in the Outpatient Diagnosis and Treatment of Bipolar Disorder in Youth," *Arch Gen Psychiatry* 64, no. 9 (September 2007): 1032–39.

11. Joyce Nolan Harrison, MD, and others, "Antipsychotic Medication Prescribing Trends in Children and Adolescents," *J Ped Health Care* 26, no. 2 (March 2012): 139–45.

12. Mark Olfson, MD, and others, "National trends in the outpatient treatment of children and adolescents with antipsychotic drugs," *Arch Gen Psychiatry* 63 (2006): 679–85.

13. Shelley Murphy, "Doctor Is Sued in Death of Girl, 4," *Boston Globe,* April 4, 2008 (accessed September 25, 2012); http://www.boston.com/news/local/articles/2008/04/04/doctor_is_sued_in_death_of_girl_4.

14. Centers for Disease Control and Prevention, "Autism Spectrum Disorders: Data and Statistics"; http://www.cdc.gov/ncbddd/autism/data.html (accessed September 4, 2012).

15. Young Shin Kim, MD, and others, "Prevalence of Autism Spectrum Disorders in a Total Population Sample," *Am J Psychiatry* 168 (2011): 904–12.

16. E. Fombonne, "Epidemiological studies of pervasive developmental disor-

ders," in F. R. Volkmar, A. Klin, R. Paul, and D. J. Cohen, eds. *Handbook of Autism and Pervasive Developmental Disorders*, 3rd ed. (Hoboken, NJ: John Wiley, 2005), 42–69.

17. Richard Horton, "A Statement by the Editors of *Lancet*," *The Lancet* 363, issue 9411 (March 6, 2004): 820–21; doi:10.1016/S0140-6736(04)15699-7.

18. A. Frances, The Autism Generation, Project Syndicate, July 19, 2011; http://www.project-syndicate.org/commentary/the-autism-generation (accessed September 19, 2012).

19. M. Ghaziuddin, "Should the *DSM V* drop Asperger syndrome?" *J Autism Dev Disord* 40 (2010): 1146–48.

20. Alan Zarendo, "Warrior Parents Fare Best in Securing Autism Services," *Los Angeles Times*, December 13, 2011, Local Section; http://www.latimes.com/news/local/autism/la-me-autism-day-two-html,0,3900437.htmlstory.

21. Christine Fountain, Alix S. Winter, and Peter S. Bearman, "Six Developmental Trajectories Characterize Children with Autism," *Pediatrics* 129, no. 5 (May 1, 2012): e1112–e1120.

22. V. Gibbs and others, "Brief Report: An Exploratory Study Comparing Diagnostic Outcomes for Autism Spectrum Disorders Under *DSM-IV*-TR with the Proposed *DSM-5* Revision," *J Autism Dev Disord* 42 (2012): 1750–56.

23. J. McPartland, B. Reichow, and F. R. Volkmar, "Sensitivity and specificity of proposed *DSM-5* diagnostic criteria for autism spectrum disorder," *Psychiatry* 51 (2012): 368–83.

24. M. Mordre, B. Groholt, A. Knudsen, E. Sponheim, A. Mykletun, and A. Myhre, "Is long term prognosis for pervasive developmental disorder not otherwise specified different from prognosis for autistic disorder? Findings from a 30 year follow up study," *Journal of Autism and Developmental Disorders* (2011); doi: 10.1007/s10803-011-1319-5.

25. M. Zimmerman and others, "Is Bipolar Disorder Overdiagnosed?" *J Clin Psychiatry* 69 (2008): 935–40.

26. A. M. Kilbourne, E. P. Post, M. S. Bauer, and others, "Therapeutic drug and cardiovascular disease risk monitoring in patients with bipolar disorder," *J Affect Disord* 102 (2007): 145–51.

27. R. C. Kessler, W. T. Chiu, O. Demler, and E. E. Walters, "Prevalence, severity, and comorbidity of twelve-month *DSM-IV* disorders in the National Comorbidity Survey Replication (NCS-R)," *Arch Gene Psychiatry* 62, no. 6 (June 2005): 617–27.

28. C. Blanco, C. Garcia, and M. R. Liebowitz, "Epidemiology of social anxiety disorder," in B. Bandelow and D. J. Stein, eds. *Social Anxiety Disorder* (New York: Marcel Dekker, 2004), 35–47.

29. Christopher Lane, PhD, *Shyness: How Normal Behavior Became a Sickness* (New Haven: Yale University Press, 2007).

30. U.S. Census Bureau Population Estimates by Demographic Characteristics. Table 2: Annual Estimates of the Population by Selected Age Groups and Sex for the United States: April 1, 2000, to July 1, 2004 (NC-EST2004-02) Source: Population Division, U.S. Census Bureau Release Date: June 9, 2005. http://www.census.gov/popest/national/asrh.

31. Gordon Parker, "Is depression overdiagnosed? Yes." *BMJ*, August 16, 2007, http://www.bmj.com/content/335/7615/328.

32. A. V. Horwitz and J. C. Wakefield, *The Loss of Sadness: How Psychiatry Transformed Normal Sorrow into Depressive Disorder* (New York: Oxford University Press, 2007).

33. Lisa K. Richardson, M.App.Psy., Christopher Frueh, PhD, and Ronald Acierno, PhD, "Prevalence Estimates of Combat-Related PTSD: A Critical Review," *Aust N Z J Psychiatry* 44, no. 1 (January 2010): 4–19.

34. PTSD and the Law: An Update http://www.google.com/url?q=http://www.ptsd.va.gov/professional/newsletters/research-quarterly/v22n1.pdf&sa=U&ei=RmxHUPWMLMusqQGCsYGICA&ved=0CBQQFjAA&usg=AFQjCNH0Vk0GP0YsK8HOvry7P2H-Dvrfng.

35. Helen Singer Kaplan, MD, *Sexual Desire Disorders: Dysfunctional Regulation of Sexual Motivation* (Levittown, PA: Brunner/Mazel, 1995).

36. Ray Moynihan, *Sex, Lies, and Pharmaceuticals: How Drug Companies Plan to Profit from Female Sexual Dysfunction* (Vancouver, BC: D & M Publishers, 2010).

37. A. Frances and M. First, "Paraphilia NOS, Nonconsent: Not Ready for the Courtroom," *Journal of American Academy of Psychiatry and the Law* 39, no. 4 (2011): 555–61.

38. S. Sreenivasan, L. E. Weinberger, and A. Frances, "Normative and Consequential Ethics in Sexually Violent Predator Evaluations," *J Amer Psychiatry and the Law* (Analysis and Commentary) 38 (2010): 386–91.

39. Robert Musil, *A Man Without Qualities* (New York: Alfred A. Knopf, 1995).

CHAPTER SIX

1. A. J. Frances, "A warning sign on the road to *DSM-V*: Beware of its unintended consequences," *Psychiatry Times* 26, no. 8 (2009): 1–4.

2. A. Frances, "Opening Pandora's Box: The Nineteen Worst Suggestions in *DSM-5*," *Psychiatric Times* (March and April 2009): http://www.psychiatrictimes.com/print/article/10168/1522341.

3. Laura Batstra and Ernst Thoutenhoofd, "The Risk That *DSM*-5 Will Further Inflate the Diagnostic Bubble," *Current Psychiatry Reviews* 8, no. 4 (November 2012): 260–63.

4. Joel Paris, MD, "The Risk That *DSM-5* Will Give Personality Dimensions a Bad Name," *Current Psychiatry Reviews* 8, no. 4 (November 2012): 268–70.

5. A. J. Frances, "Dimensional diagnosis of personality—not whether, but when and which," *Psychol Inq* 4 (1993): 110–11.

6. Dayle K. Jones, PhD, "The Risk That *DSM-5* Will Reduce the Credibility of Psychiatric Diagnosis," *Current Psychiatry Reviews* 8, no. 4 (November 2012): 277–80.

7. A. Frances, "Whither DSM-5," *British Journal of Psychiatry* 195, no. 5 (November 2009): 391–92.

8. A. Frances, "The First Draft of DSM-V," *British Journal of Psychiatry, March 2, 2010, http://www.bmj.com/content/340/bmj.c1168?tab=responses.

9. James Phillips, MD, and Allen Frances, MD, "The Seven Biggest Risks Posed by *DSM-5*," *Current Psychiatry Reviews* 8, no. 4 (November 2012): 257–59.

10. Dayle K. Jones, "A Critique of the *DSM-5* Field Trials," *Journal of Nervous & Mental Disease* 200, no. 6 (June 2012): 517–19; doi: 10.1097/NMD.0b013e318257c699.

11. A. Frances, "Limitations of Field Trials," *American Journal of Psychiatry* 166, no. 12 (December 2009): 1322.

12. Martin Whitely and Melissa Raven, PhD, "The Risk that *DSM-5* Will Result in a Misallocation of Scarce Resources," *Current Psychiatry Reviews* 8, no. 4 (November 2012): 281–86.

13. Gary Greenberg, PhD, "The Risk That *DSM-5* Will Affect the Way We See Ourselves," *Current Psychiatry Reviews* 8, no. 4 (November 2012): 287–89.

14. F. Leibenluft and others. "Chronic vs. episodic irritability in youth: A community-based, longitudinal study of clinical and diagnostic associations," *Journal of Child and Adolescent Psychopharmacology* 16 (2006): 456–66.

15. S. Crystal, M. Olfson, C. Huang, H. Pincus, and T. Gerard, "Broadened use of atypical antipsychotics: Safety, effectiveness, and policy changes," *Health Affairs* 28, no. 5 (2009): 770–81.

16. Bradley T. Hyman and others, "National Institute on Aging–Alzheimer's Association guidelines for the neuropathologic assessment of Alzheimer's disease," *Alzheimer's & Dementia: The Journal of the Alzheimer's Association* 8, no. 1 (2012): 1–13.

17. L. M. Schwartz and S. Woloshin, "How the FDA forgot the evidence: the case of donepezil 23 mg," *BMJ* 344 (2012): 1086.

18. Worst Pills, Best Pills, "Aricept," *Public Citizen,* September 2012 (accessed September 5, 2012); https://www.worstpills.org/results.cfm?drug_id=217&x=34&y=6.

19. Ethical Issues in Diagnosing and Treating Alzheimer's Disease; http://www.ncbi.nlm.nih.gov/pmc/articles/PMC2990623.

20. J. I. Hudson, E. Hiripi, H. G. Pope Jr., and R. C. Kessler "The Prevalence and Correlates of Eating Disorders in the National Comorbidity Survey Replication," *Biological Psychiatry* 61, no. 3 (2007): 348–58.

21. Joanna Moncrief and Sami Timimi, "Critical analysis of the concept of adult attention-deficit hyperactivity disorder," *The Psychiatrist* 35 (2011): 334–38; doi: 10.1192/pb.bp.110.033423.

22. A. G. Harrison, M. J. Edwards, and K. C. Parker, "Identifying students faking ADHD: Preliminary findings and strategies for detection," *Archives of Clinical Neuropsychology* 22, no. 5 (2007): 577–88.

23. C. A. Quinn, "Detection of malingering in assessment of adult ADHD," *Archives of Clinical Neuropsychology* 18, no. 4 (2003): 379–95.

24. B. K. Sullivan, K. May, and L. Galbally, "Symptom exaggeration by college adults in attention-deficit hyperactivity disorder and learning disorder assessments," *Applied Neuropsychology* 14, no. 3 (2007): 189–207.

25. Jerome C. Wakefield and Mark F. Schmitz, "Recurrence of Depression After Bereavement-Related Depression: Evidence for the Validity of *DSM-IV* Bereavement Exclusion from the Epidemiologic Catchment Area Study," *Journal of Nervous & Mental Disease* 200, no. 6 (June 2012): 480–85; doi: 10.1097/NMD.0b013e318248213f.

26. "Living with Grief" (editorial) *Lancet* 379, no. 9816 (18 February 2012): 589. doi: 10.1016/S01406736(12)60248-7.

27. Arthur Kleinman, "Culture, Bereavement, and Psychiatry," *The Lancet* 379, issue 9816 (February 18, 2012): 608–609, doi:10.1016/S0140-6736(12)60258-X.

28. Richard A. Friedman, MD, "Grief, Depression, and the *DSM-5*," *N Engl J Med* 366 (May 17, 2012): 1855–57.

29. Joanne Cacciatore, "Blog Post Goes Viral: MISS Foundation + Over 75K Readers Denounce *DSM-5* Changes to Bereavement Exclusion," PR Web, posted March 6, 2012; http://www.prweb.com/releases/DSMV_EthicalRelativism/Cacciatore/prweb9258619.htm (accessed September 5, 2012).

30. Ron Mihordin, "Behavioral Addiction—Quo Vadis?" *Journal of Nervous & Mental Disease* 200, no. 6 (June 2012): 489–91; doi: 10.1097/NMD.0b013e318257c503.

31. R. Collier, "Internet addiction: New-age diagnosis or symptom of age-old problem?" *Canadian Medical Association Journal* 181, no. 9 (2009): 575–76.

32. Wikipedia. "Oniomania," last modified Auguat 4, 2012; http://en.wikipedia.org/wiki/Oniomania.

33. Wikipedia. "Workaholic," last modified August 22, 2012; http://en.wikipedia.org/wiki/Workaholism.

34. Wikipedia, "Exercise Addiction," lasted modified June 29, 2012; http://en.wikipedia.org/wiki/Exercise_addiction.

35. Wikipedia, "Tanning Addiction," last modified August 2, 2012; http://en.wikipedia.org/wiki/Tanning_addiction.

36. Jane Collingwood, "Does Chocolate Addiction Exist?" PsychCentral.com, http://psychcentral.com/lib/2006/does-chocolate-addiction-exist.

37. Alison Yung, MD, "Should attenuated psychosis syndrome be included in *DSM-5*?" *The Lancet* 379, issue 9816 (February 18, 2012): 591–92; doi:10.1016/S0140-6736(11)61507-9.

38. Peter J. Weiden, MD, "The Risk That *DSM*-5 Will Promote Even More Inappropriate Anti-psychotic Exposure in Children and Teenagers," *Current Psychiatry Reviews* 8, no. 4 (November 2012): 271–76.

39. C. M. Corcoran, M. B. First, and B. Cornblatt, "The psychosis risk syndrome and its proposed inclusion in the *DSM-V*: A risk-benefit analysis," *Schizophr Res* 120 (2010): 16–22.

40. Colin Ross "*DSM-5* and the 'Psychosis Risk Syndrome': Eight reasons to reject it," *Psychosis: Psychological, Social and Integrative Approaches* 2, no. 2 (2010): 107–10; http://www.tandfonline.com/doi/abs/10.1080/17522431003763323.

41. A. Jennex and D. M. Gardner, "Monitoring and management of metabolic risk factors in outpatients taking antipsychotic drugs: a controlled study," *Can J Psychiatry* 53 (2008): 4–42.

42. Neeltje M. Batelaan, Jan Spijker, Ron de Graaf, and Cuijpers, "Mixed Anxiety Depression Should Not Be Included in *DSM-5*," *Pim Journal of Nervous & Mental Disease* 200, no. 6 (June 2012): 495–98; doi: 10.1097/NMD.0b013e318257c4c9.

43. K. Walters and others, "Mixed anxiety and depressive disorder outcomes: prospective cohort study in primary care," *Br J Psychiatry* 198, no. 6 (June 2011): 472–78.

44. A. J. Frances, "The forensic risks of *DSM-V* and how to avoid them," *J Am Acad Psychiatry Law* 38 (2010): 11–14.

45. P. Good and J. Burstein, "Hebephilia and the Construction of a Fictitious Diagnosis," *Journal of Nervous & Mental Disease* 200, no. 6 (June 2012): 492–94; doi: 10.1097/NMD.0b013e318257c4f1.

46. Allen Frances, MD, "The Risk That *DSM-5* Will Exacerbate the SVP Mess in Forensic Psychiatry," *Current Psychiatry Reviews* 8, no. 4 (November 2012): 264–67.

47. A. J. Reid Finlayson, John Sealy, and Peter R. Martin, "Sexual Addiction and Compulsivity," *Journal of Treatment & Prevention* 8, no. 3–4 (2001): 241–51; doi:10.1080/107201601753459946.

48. R. C. Kessler, K. R. Merikangas, P. Berglind, W. W. Eaton, D. S. Koretz, and E. E. Walters, "Mild disorders should not be eliminated from the DSM-5," *Arch Gen Psychiatry* 60 (2003): 1117–22.

CHAPTER SEVEN

1. Mark Thornton, "Alcohol Prohibition Was a Failure," Policy Analysis (1991); http://www.cato.org/publications/policy-analysis/alcohol-prohibition-was-failure.

2. "The Drug War Spreads Instability," *The Globe and Mail*, April 26, 2012, last updated September 6, 2012, Editorial Section; http://www.theglobeandmail.com/commentary/the-drug-war-spreads-instability/article4104311.

3. Centers for Disease Control and Prevention, "Prescription Painkiller Overdoses at Epidemic Levels,"(2011); http://www.cdc.gov/media/releases/2011/p1101_flu_pain_killer_overdose.html.

4. Global Commission on Drug Policy, "The War on Drugs and HIV/AIDS: How the Criminalization of Drug Use Fuels the Global Pandemic," http://globalcommissionondrugs.org/wp-content/themes/gcdp_v1/pdf/GCDP_HIV-AIDS_2012_REFERENCE.pdf.

5. Melissa Raven, "Direct-to-Consumer Advertising: Healthy Education or Corporate Spin?" Healthy Skepticism International News (2004); http://www.healthyskepticism.org/global/news/int/hsin2004-09.

6. Lee Fang, "When a Congressman Becomes a Lobbyist, He Gets a 1,452 Percent Raise (on Average)," *The Nation*, March 24, 2012. http://www.thenation.com/article/166809/when-congressman-becomes-lobbyist-he-gets-1452-percent-raise-average#.

7. Marcia Angell, "The Truth About the Drug Companies," *New York Review of Books* 51, no. 12 (2004): 52–58.

8. K. Abbasi and R. Smith, "No More Free Lunches," *BMJ* 326, no. 7400 (2003): 1155.

9. A. Fugh-Berman and S. Ahari, "Following the Script: How Drug Reps Make Friends and Influence Doctors," *PLoS Med* 4, no. 4 (2007), http://www.ncbi.nlm.nih.gov/pubmed/17455991.

10. "An Unhealthy Disregard," *Nat Med* 16, no. 6 (2010): 609.

11. R. N. Moynihan, "Kissing Goodbye to Key Opinion Leaders," *Med J Aust* 196, no. 11 (2012): 671.

12. John Kaplan, "The Cost of Doing Business? Pharmaceutical Company Fines," Bioethics Today, August 2, 2012, http://www.amc.edu/bioethicsblog/post.cfm/the-cost-of-doing-business-pharmaceutical-company-fines.

13. B. Mintzes, "Should Patient Groups Accept Money from Drug Companies? No," *BMJ* 334, no. 7600 (2007): 935.

14. B. Mintzes, "Disease Mongering in Drug Promotion: Do Governments Have a Regulatory Role?" *PLoS Med* 3, no. 4 (2006); http://www.plosmedicine.org/article/info%3Adoi%2F10.1371%2Fjournal.pmed.0030198.

15. A. J. Fyer and others, "Discontinuation of Alprazolam Treatment in Panic Patients," *Am J Psychiatry* 144, no. 3 (1987): 303–308.

16. David Rosenfeld, "Jackson Case Highlights Medical Ethics," *Pacific Standard* (2012) http://www.psmag.com/health/jackson-case-highlights-medical-ethics-3572/

17. L. Batstra and A. Frances, "Diagnostic Inflation: Causes and a Suggested Cure," *J Nerv Ment Dis* 200, no. 6 (2012): 474–79.

18. J. S. Comer, M. Olfson, and R. Mojtabai, "National Trends in Child and Adolescent Psychotropic Polypharmacy in Office-Based Practice, 1996–2007," *J Am Acad Child Adolesc Psychiatry* 49, no. 10 (2010): 1001–10.

19. E. R. Hajjar, A. C. Cafiero, and J. T. Hanlon, "Polypharmacy in Elderly Patients," *Am J Geriatr Pharmacother* 5, no. 4 (2007): 345–51.

20. V. Barbour and others, "False Hopes, Unwarranted Fears: The Trouble with Medical News Stories," *PLoS Med* 5, no. 5 (2008) http://www.plosmedicine.org/article/info%3Adoi%2F10.1371%2Fjournal.pmed.0050118,

CHAPTER EIGHT

1. A. Frances, *Essentials of Psychiatric Diagnosis* (New York: Guilford Press, 2013).

INDEX

ABOUT THE AUTHOR

ALLEN FRANCES, M.D., was the chairman of the *DSM-IV* Task Force and part of the leadership group for *DSM-III* and *DSM-III-R*. He is a professor emeritus and former chair of the Department of Psychiatry and Behavioral Science at Duke University School of Medicine. He lives in Coronado, California, and travels and lectures extensively worldwide.